Burnout Among Social Workers

Burnout Among Social Workers

David F. Gillespie
Editor

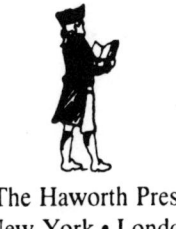

The Haworth Press
New York • London

Burnout Among Social Workers has also been published as *Journal of Social Service Research,* Volume 10, Number 1, Fall 1986.

© 1987 by The Haworth Press, Inc. All rights reserved. No part of this book may be reproduced or utilized in any form or by any means, electronic or mechanical, including photocopying, microfilm and recording, or by any information storage and retrieval system, without permission in writing from the publisher. Printed in the United States of America.

The Haworth Press, Inc., 12 West 32 Street, New York, NY 10001
EUROSPAN/Haworth, 3 Henrietta Street, London WC2E 8LU England

Library of Congress Cataloging-in-Publication Data

Burnout among social workers.

    Has also been published as Journal of social service research, v. 10, no. 1, 1986.
    Includes bibliographies. 1. Social Workers United States Job Stress. 2. Burn out (Psychology) I. Gillespie, David F.
HV10.5.B867   1987   361.3'01'9   87-14930
ISBN 0-86656-666-X

Burnout Among Social Workers

CONTENTS

Preface	1
David F. Gillespie	
Introduction	3
David F. Gillespie	
An Approach to the Study of Burnout in Professional Care Providers in Human Service Organizations	7
Myrna M. Courage	
David D. Williams	
Linear Model	10
Multidimensional Model	11
Implications	19
Factors Associated with Burnout in the Social Services: An Exploratory Study	23
Craig Winston LeCroy	
Mark R. Rank	
Review of the Literature	24
Method	26
Results	29
Conclusion	36
Gender Differences in Work Stress Among Clinical Social Workers	41
David P. Himle	
Srinika D. Jayaratne	
Wayne A. Chess	
The Sample	42
Study Variables	43
Results	46
Discussion	52

The Association of Burnout and Social Work Practitioners' Impressions of Their Clients: Empirical Evidence   **57**
    Kevin J. Corcoran

Method	59
Results and Discussion	61
Conclusions	64

Social Workers and Burnout: A Psychological Description   **67**
    Mary Johnson
    Gerald L. Stone

Method	68
Results	71
Discussion	75

Burnout Among Social Workers Working with Physically Disabled Persons and Bereaved Families   **81**
    Ariela Stav
    Victor Florian
    Esther Zernitsky Shurka

Method	84
Results	87
Discussion	90

Burnout Research in the Social Services: A Critique   **95**
    Christina Maslach

Contributions of the Special Issue	96
Shortcomings of the Special Issue	98
Concluding Remarks	104

Burnout Among Social Workers

Preface

The road to publishing this special issue has been a twisting and winding one, with numerous delays, misplaced directional signs, potholes, and precipitous inclines and declines. The project was conceived in the Spring of 1983 when there was a lot of talk about empirical research on burnout, and it seemed feasible that a collection of empirical studies could be brought together as a state of the art review representing the first ten years of work since Freudenberger (1974) adapted the term. The idea was to assemble a set of studies which would reflect the developing state of empirical knowledge regarding burnout. We planned to announce the special issue in the 1983 autumn issue of JSSR, receive and review articles throughout 1984, and then publish the issue in 1985 as a ten-year benchmark collection.

The special issue was a good idea, and the plan to build it was rational. Like many plans, however, implementation introduced a number of complications. First, the announcement scheduled to appear in the Autumn 1983 issue did not appear until the Spring issue of 1984 which, to further complicate matters, was distributed about mid-year. This made it necessary to extend the review period.

Second, extending the review period was also necessary because too few manuscripts were submitted in response to the announcement. A few empirically based articles were submitted, and an even larger number of non-empirical review pieces were submitted. This development was consistent with previous independent assessments by Maslach (1982) and Gillespie (1983) which found work with the concept of burnout to be largely anecdotal and non-empirical. Apparently, much of the talk about research on burnout has been wishful thinking. It is significant, therefore, to have achieved the collection of empirically based articles brought together in this special issue. We hope the work here portends a model for the immediate future.

Third, the original plan contracted co-equal editing of the special issue by David Gillespie and Christina Maslach. But, as it turned out, the extended review period collided with a sabbatical that took Maslach out of the country during the time that manuscripts were being reviewed. Because of the timing, it became necessary to make commitments to publish prior to Maslach's reviewing the manuscripts. To deal with this problem, standard JSSR procedures involving anonymous reviewers were used. In addition, it was decided that the issue would be strengthened if Maslach assumed the role of discussant rather than co-editor. This made it possible for her to offer a candid overview, assessing each of the contributions and their collective significance. Maslach's role as critic is particularly powerful, not only because of her seminal work in the field, but also because each of the empirically based articles in this special issue used the Maslach Burnout Inventory (MBI) in their studies.

DFG

REFERENCES

Freudenberger, Herbert J. (#1, 1974). Staff Burnout. *Journal of Social Issues* 30(1), 159-165.

Gillespie, David F. (1983). *Understanding and Combatting Burnout*. Monticello, IL: Vance Bibliographies.

Maslach, Christina (1982). *Burnout: The Cost of Caring*. Englewood Cliffs, NJ: Prentice-Hall.

Introduction

The idea of burnout has attracted considerable attention. It has been noted among a wide range of professionals: social workers, teachers, business executives, dentists, police, department store managers, psychotherapists, lawyers, day care workers, nurses, and others. Essays and articles have appeared in dozens of popular magazines. Short articles on burnout have appeared in many newspapers. Although the word "burnout" in the popular media lacks precision, the recognition and interest shown in the problem suggest its relevance in contemporary society.

Scholarly work with the concept of burnout has progressed more slowly than public interest, but a research base is evolving and there are increasing numbers of professionals and researchers from different intellectual backgrounds reading one another's work to learn more about burnout, its distribution in different occupational groups, and ways of reducing the problem. There have been several hundred articles published in professional journals. Some of these articles deal with occupational stress or other phenomena related to burnout, but many of them focus explicitly on the concept of burnout.

While burnout continues to be presented as a stress-related concept, there are many who make a sharp distinction between burnout and other stress research. People working with the concept of burnout are beginning to refer to it as an area or sub-field. This is an interesting development because it is not an area of research that is dominated by any one discipline, although there are probably more psychologists than any other discipline currently working in the area. Over twenty dissertations have been written on burnout, and more are on the way. It seems that despite its popularity the notion of burnout has been accepted as a potentially meaningful scientific concept. The initial flurry of interest, therefore, will probably settle down into more systematic inquiries and theory building. This is already evident in the transition from case study methods to broader based surveys, and field experiments.

The exceptionally diverse and rapidly expanding body of literature on burnout suggests the need for empirical assessments. Work on burnout cuts across psychology, sociology, social work, medicine, education, administration or management, and others dealing with human service professionals. This wide scope of work with burnout is both a strength and weakness. It is a strength in that the biases and limitations of knowledge tend to be captured in the assumptions and orientations of particular fields; and often the biases or limitations of one field are the strong points of a different field. In this sense, the interdisciplinary nature of the emerging field of burnout can be recognized as a strong asset.

The weakness with interdisciplinary approaches is that communication between different disciplines is difficult due to dissimilar assumptions and special jargon, and also because the ideas and findings regarding a given phenomenon like burnout are published in widely scattered journals representing the variety of disciplines concerned with the topic. Although there have been some recent literature reviews and bibliographies on burnout, these serve only to direct one through the maze of fields to particular articles.

Drawing together empirical articles on burnout helps to identify and discuss areas of agreement and disagreement, and in so doing provide the basis for a more concerted effort. The seven articles contained in this issue include a think piece, five empirical studies, and a critique. The think piece by Courage and Williams presents an approach to theory by conceptualizing potentially important variables as attributes of (a) professionals, (b) the organizations they work in, and (c) the clients they serve. This approach begins to set the stage for theory by focusing on processes of interaction between dimensions of the three clustered blocks of variables. Thinking about dynamic patterns of association between sets of variables describing professionals and clients in the context of organizations is admittedly difficult. But it seems clear that complex phenomena like burnout require theory to be understood. Practice without theory makes problems impregnable.

LeCroy and Rank report on 106 social workers from agencies in two midwestern towns of two different states. They assess the influence of demographic, psychological, and job situation variables on burnout. Their data support Maslach's (1978) claim that burnout results more from job situations than personality factors. A hypothesis concerning the personality factor of assertiveness is not supported, while four job variables—professional self-esteem, work autonomy, discrepancy between present attainment and aspirations, and salary—are associated significantly with burnout. Regression analysis shows the discrepancy variable to be particularly strong.

Corcoran studied 88 female members of the Texas Chapter of NASW. Consistent with previous work, age and experience were found to be associated negatively with burnout; older and more experienced social workers are less likely to burnout. Two dimensions of the MBI—emotional exhaustion and depersonalization—were associated significantly with social workers' impressions of their clients. Social workers with high levels of burnout revealed negative impressions of their clients. It is clear from these data that burnout affects clinical practice.

Himle, Jayaratne, and Chess studied a sample of 617 clinical social workers drawn from the national membership list of NASW. Gender differences are assessed for relationships of job situation and personality variables with burnout. Low levels of emotional support from supervisors and co-workers is associated with burnout for females, but not for males. Increased contact with clients is associated with decreased personal accomplishment for women, but increased personal accomplishment for men. Decreased role ambiguity is associated with increased personal accomplishment for women, while decreased role ambiguity is associated with increased depersonalization for men. Increased job comfort is associated with a greater sense of personal accomplishment for women only. The interpretations given for these gender differences sharpen and clarify hypothesized processes underlying burnout.

Johnson and Stone studied 46 social workers in county social service agencies of the upper midwest. Burnout is associated with higher levels of relatively unpleasant events ("hassles" or irritations) which characterize daily living, such as not liking work duties, not having enough time for family, not getting enough rest, etcetera. They also report a significant positive association between Type A behavior patterns—competitiveness, impatience, easy provocation, excessive drive and hostility—and feelings of personal accomplishment. Most of the work on Type A personalities has documented negative effects. The importance of this work, therefore, relates primarily to the potential cross-fertilization of work on burnout with work on Type A personalities and self-efficacy.

Stav, Florian, and Shurka studied 112 female social workers drawn from both rehabilitation and social welfare agencies in Israel. Social workers in the welfare agencies use a generic approach to deal with a wide range of problems, while those providing rehabilitation services function in a more limited fashion in highly centralized bureaucracies. The rehabilitation workers have higher burnout scores than the welfare workers on the personal involvement dimension. Burnout scores are lower than those reported for American samples, but similar associations between variables is demonstrated. The different organizational settings, however, influence the way variables such as caseload, time for staff consultation, time for job supervision, satisfaction with supervision, and bureaucratic intervention relate to burnout.

Maslach critiques each article to assess the contributions of this special issue. She reviews problems with definitions, atheoretical orientations, and overall "conceptual fuzziness" which has plagued research on burnout from the beginning. The need to move forward with more representative samples such as those drawn by Himle et al. and Stav et al. is discussed. The importance of measurement is heavily stressed. Proper referencing, accurate description, adherence to exact procedures of operationalization for a given measure, and the use of different measures are essential to adequate knowledge development. A well-placed caution about causal inferences from cross-sectional data is advanced, along with a call for longitudinal research. Noting that "systematic research on burnout has gotten underway only recently," Maslach refers to this special issue as "a landmark event" which "may serve as a model for future studies."

DFG

An Approach to the Study of Burnout in Professional Care Providers in Human Service Organizations

Myrna M. Courage
David D. Williams

SUMMARY. A multidimensional approach is proposed for the study of burnout in professional care providers. The approach depicts relationships between care provider, human service organization and recipient of care in the development of burnout in the providers of human services. This article is both a literature review and a description of a new conceptualization based on, but not limited to, existing literature.

Burnout is emerging as the occupational hazard of the helping professions. The burnout syndrome results from intensive contact with people who need help. According to the literature, care providers are at risk for burnout when the recipient of care presents with problems in which either the chronicity, complexity, or acuity of the client's needs are beyond the resources of the care provider or the human service organization.

This paper presents a conceptual model for the study of the relationship between the occurrence of burnout in care providers, the human service organization, and the recipient of care. The

---

Ms. Courage is Assistant Professor, College of Nursing, University of Florida in Gainesville, and is a doctoral student in social work at Florida State University in Tallahassee. Dr. Williams is Associate Professor, College of Nursing, University of Florida, Gainesville, and is a care provider in Alachua County Organization for Rural Needs. Requests for reprints should be addressed to Ms. Courage. The authors would like to thank Dr. Beverly Henry for reviewing a previous draft of the manuscript.

© 1987 by The Haworth Press, Inc. All rights reserved.

care provider, the human service organization and the recipient of care are identified as essential components of the human services delivery system. What is proposed is a model by which the variables of each of the components may be identified in relationship to variables associated with each of the other two components of the system. Thus the model provides for the simultaneous identification of variables postulated as contributing to the development of burnout in care providers.

Burnout refers to a syndrome which occurs in the care provider as a response to chronic emotional stress and which arises from the social interaction between a care provider and the recipient of care. The research of Berkeley Planning Associates (1977), Maslach and Jackson (1981) and Perlman and Hartman (1982) provides support for conceptualizing burnout as emotional and physical exhaustion, reduced personal productivity, and a sense of depersonalization.

The literature describes two major categories of variables related to burnout in care providers. The categories pertain to the care provider and the human service organization as the workplace. The provision of care takes place within the context of the helping relationship. The essence of the helping relationship is a meaningful involvement with another that includes an investment of one's resources for the care of another. According to Maslach (1982) the constant expenditure of energy on behalf of others creates a pattern of emotional overload that results in emotional and physical exhaustion of the care provider. The emotionally and physically exhausted care provider is no longer able to maintain the involvement expected in a helping relationship.

Maslach's description of burnout assumes an association between burnout and the direct contact with clients having constant and intensive needs. Although there is little research that explores the characteristics of this relationship, Berglund and Permelia (1979) found the rates of emotional exhaustion of care providers in mental hospitals increased with the number of hours spent in direct patient contact.

The client who seeks assistance from the human service organization has expectations as to the needed services. The care provider similarly has expectations as to his or her capabilities in providing care. When the relationship between the care provider and the recipient of care achieves neither the recipient's expectations nor the expected outcomes of the care provider, culpability may be assigned to either (Maslach, 1982). In the literature, culpability is most frequently assigned to personality traits of care providers. Freudenberger (1975) described the personality type susceptible to burnout as the over-dedicated and over-committed worker. Further support is provided by Edelwich and Brodsky (1980), who describe burnout as associated with the over commitment of the young, enthused care provider. Specific personality traits associated with burnout in the care provider include non-assertiveness in dealing with people, impatience, intolerance in confronting obstacles, and lack of self-confidence (Gann, 1979; Hasenfeld, 1983). A restricted social life with all meaning and gratification derived from work is another personality attribute associated with burnout (Freudenberger, 1980).

The work context has also been associated with the development of burnout (Gillespie, 1981). The work context defines some of the parameters for contact between the care provider and the recipient of care. The availability and allocation of resources, the definition of organizational goals, and the determination of eligibility for care are also defined by the work context. The organizational structure determines the communication and interactional patterns among care providers and between care providers and recipients of care.

Quantity of the work load, the availability of a supportive environment, and the ability to mobilize resources for the provision of services emerge from the literature as contributing factors to burnout within the work setting. Case load size is the most frequently identified organizational variable associated with burnout (Berkeley Planning Associates, 1977; Freudenberger, 1980; Larson, Gilbertson & Powell, 1978; Perlman & Hartman, 1982; Soloman, 1979). A large case size contributes to work overload, thereby taxing the resources of the care provider and thus potentiating burnout. In addition, the organizational components of leadership, communication, supervision and responsibility have been identified as factors contributing to burnout (Berkeley Planning Associates, 1977).

Social and physical isolation in the work setting is another variable identified with burnout. Isolation may arise from the demands of the work load, peer conflict, competition, and lack of rapport, all of which interfere with collegial support and interactions (Larson, Gilbertson & Powell, 1978). In addition, the physical structure of the work setting may isolate the care providers from support systems (Maslach, 1982). Task significance and productivity have been found to be significantly related to burnout (Maslach & Jackson, 1981). Care providers in human service organizations who expect to make a meaningful contribution to others through the provision of services tend to be vulnerable to burnout when expectations are not fulfilled. Minimal input into policy decisions and inflexible institutional roles were the organizational variables Maslach identified as associated with burnout.

LINEAR MODEL

Conceptual models have been developed to identify the relationship between the variables associated with the burnout syndrome. Perlman and Hartman (1982) present a model based upon the previous work of House and Wells (1978). The model presents a linear progression of four stages of stress, including situation, perception, response and outcome. Each stage relates to a set of personal variables and a set of organizational variables. For example, the first stage of stress describes the degree to which a situation is conducive to stress. This stage is related to the personal variables of ability, time, family demands, and expectations, and to the organizational variables of work load, expected performance, and role ambiguity.

According to the model, stress culminates in burnout in the fourth stage. Using the model, each set of variables functions as a discrete entity impacting with only one of the stages of stress development. For example, the personal variable of tolerance for ambiguity is pivotal between the first stage of stress (that is, degree to which the situation is conducive to stress) and the second stage (level of perceived stress). However, tolerance for ambiguity is not conceptualized as interacting with other personal variables such as physical health or professional identity. Physical health and professional identity are conceptualized as pivotal between the second and third stage of stress. In reality, poor physical health or professional role ambiguity could be the cause of initial stress rather than impinging only on later stages as suggested by the model. The model implies an additive, invariant sequence of events leading to burnout. Conceptualizing personal variables and organizational variables as discrete entities impacting on specific stages of stress may be an oversimplification of the actual dynamics of burnout. The sequencing of the consecutive stages of stress, with the alignment of discrete variables according to a specific stage of stress, implies an isolated impact and a temporal ordering of events leading to the development of each stage of burnout. According to this model, increased stress could be prevented through alteration of a specific variable only at a specific stage. However, no experimental evidence exists to support the sequential impact of personal and organizational variables on the development of burnout in care providers. The simultaneous impact of multiple variables may be more devastating, and this view is congruent with the cumulative effect of stress documented in the literature.

In human service organizations the recipient of care adds a third dimension that impacts on both the organization and the care provider. For example, recipients of care are self-activating entities who define their own needs (Larson, Gilbertson & Powell, 1978) and create demands for the expertise and services of the care providers and for the resources of the human service organization. The complexity and acuity of human needs create additional stresses for the care provider and the organization. Consequently, a realistic conceptualization of burnout must consider the additional relationship between the characteristics of the recipients' needs and the variables associated with both the care provider and the organization.

MULTIDIMENSIONAL MODEL

The model in Figure 1 provides a schematic representation of the proposed relationships among the variables associated with the provider of care, the organization, and the recipient of care, as they contribute to the development of burnout. The model is conceptualized as a cube consisting of smaller cubes or cells. The

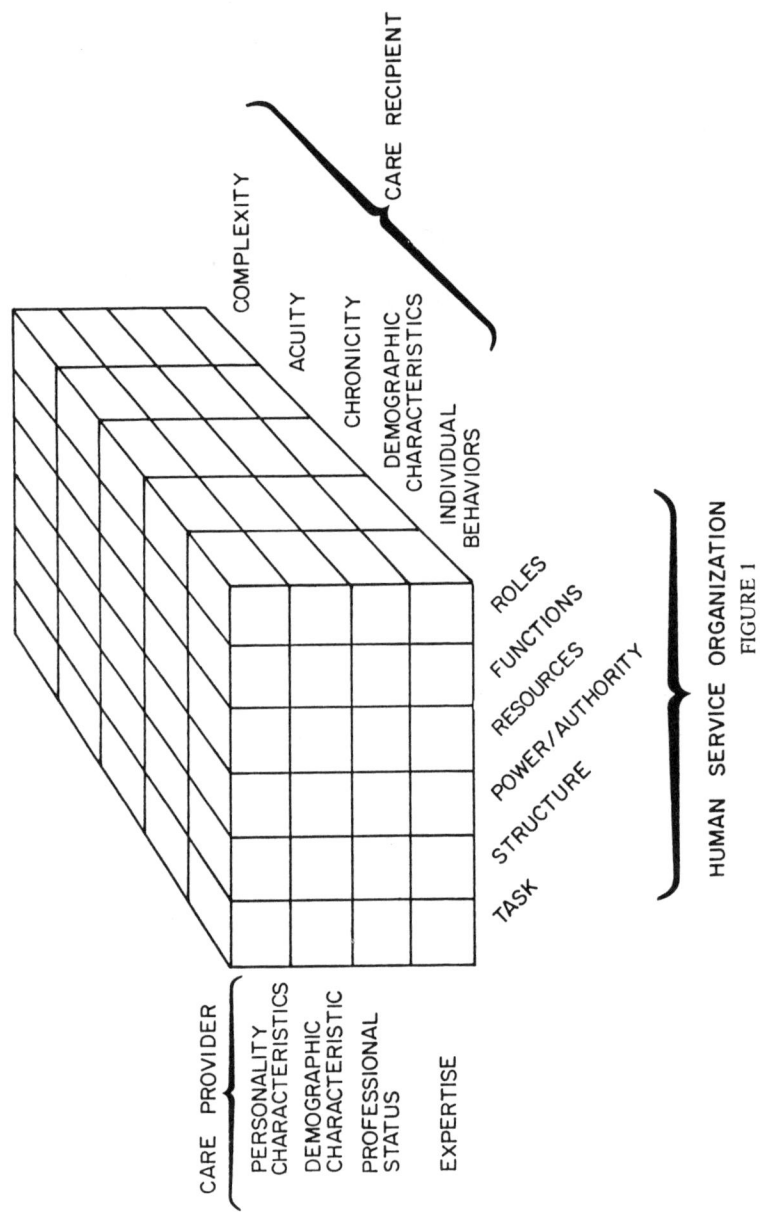

HUMAN SERVICE ORGANIZATION
FIGURE 1

three axes of the cube represent variables associated with the care provider, organization, and recipient of care. Each cell proposes an association with one of the variables from each axis.

Care Provider

The axis representing the care provider includes characteristics of individual personality, demographic characteristics, professional status, and expertise variables.

Personality characteristics. Personality variables refer to the personal characteristics that may render the care provider susceptible to burnout and include the degree to which the care provider is committed to and involved with helping people. Burnout in care providers has been associated with the personality characteristics of being empathetic, idealistic, altruistic, and over-committed in the service of others to the detriment of self (Freudenberger, 1975; Gann, 1979; House, 1981). A personality profile of those susceptible to burnout has been constructed using characteristics such as unassertiveness, impatience, intolerance, submissiveness, fearfulness and inability to establish limits within the helping relationship (Edelwich & Brodsky, 1980; Freudenberger, 1980; Gann, 1979; Hasenfeld, 1983; Pines, Aronson & Kafry, 1981). The combination of personality characteristics that render the individual care provider vulnerable to self-depletion in the service of others leads to burnout.

Demographic characteristics. Demographic variables that have been associated with burnout include age, marital and family status, and education. Younger care providers are more susceptible to burnout than their older counterparts (Freudenberger, 1980; Heckman, 1981; Maslach, 1982). Single care providers tend to be at greater risk for burnout than divorced care providers, and both single and divorced care providers tend to be at greater risk than married care providers (Maslach, 1982). Although education has been associated with the occurrence of burnout in care providers, education without practical experience tends to create the greatest discrepancies between idealistic expectation for service and the realities of the human service organization and renders the care provider most vulnerable to burnout (Corcoran & Bryce, 1983; Maslach, 1982). Education in care providers has been associated with individual burnout in human service organizations (Edelwich & Brodsky, 1980).

Professional status. The care provider in the human service organization is usually a member of a professional organization. The professional status of the care provider implies the adherence to the standards of that profession and the autonomy to practice within legal and professional parameters (Steers, 1977). On the other hand, the human service organization also defines the parameters for the provision of care (Hall, 1982; Perrow, 1979). Consequently, conflict between expectations of the service organization and the professional organization creates stress which contributes to the development of burnout.

Expertise. The expertise of the care provider is essential to meet the expectations of the care recipient and the human service organization. Given the indeterminant technology of human services (Hasenfeld, 1983) and the intractability of human problems (Weiner, 1982), there may be ambiguity about the degree and kind of expertise required of the care provider. The degree to which the expectations of both the care recipient and the human service organization exceed the actual expertise of the care provider is a significant factor contributing to the development of burnout.

Human Service Organizations

The axis representing the human service organization includes tasks, structure, power/authority, resources, functions, and role variables.

Task variables. Task variables are associated with the organization's unit of work. Burnout has been shown to be related to work overload, the significance of the work performed, and the work context which includes the type and amount of contact with care recipients and between care providers (Daley, 1979; Edelwich & Brodsky, 1980; Larson, Gilbertson & Powell, 1978; Maslach, 1982; Warshaw, 1979). The nature of the task determines the amount of energy expenditure required to perform the task. The extent to which the task requires intense and repeated involvement with people increases the energy expenditure and the risk of burnout.

Structure. The structure of the human service organization determines the relationships between the workers and the type and amount of interaction between care recipients, care providers, and supervisors. The organization may follow a bureaucratic model with clearly defined authority structure, division of labor, and formalized rules and channels of communication, or the organization may follow a contingency model where authority, people and resources are allocated according to task (Weiner, 1982). To the extent that the organizational structure is flexible enough to accommodate the unique and changing needs of the care recipient and provider, the structure is supportive to the care provider. To the extent that the organizational structure lacks the flexibility to meet human needs, the care provider is at risk for burnout (Maslach, 1982; Pines, Aronson & Kafry, 1981).

Power/authority. The organization makes provisions for the distribution of power and authority. Authority refers to the degree to which care providers have decision making rights (Hasenfeld, 1983; Sutton & Ford, 1982). Specifically in human service organizations, authority is the right to make decisions that guide the actions of the care recipients (Hasenfeld, 1983). In human service organizations, the care recipient retains an element of power in decisions related to his care. In fact, the care provider may function in a consultant role and the care recipient may retain all power concerning the decisions about his care. Lacking a sense of impact in the decision making structure, the care provider may perceive an inability to effect outcome (Pines, Aronson & Kafry, 1981). An additional factor contributing to burnout in care providers may be the shared authority that emerges in the interagency model often required for the delivery of human services. The interagency model further limits the ability of the care provider to control outcomes, adding to actual loss of autonomy.

Resources. The human service organization is dependent upon the environment for the resources to maintain service delivery (Hasenfeld, 1983). The resources provided by the environment may be inadequate to meet either the service goals of the organization or the requirements or demands of the care recipients. The general inadequacy of resources to maintain the quality of service expected by the care provider and by the care recipient may be a factor in the occurrence of burnout in care providers. In addition, the paucity of resources may require the care provider to actively negotiate for the limited resources, establishing a competitive atmosphere and the demise of the collegial relationships essential to buffer the effect of work stress (Cooper & Payne, 1980; House, 1981). In a limited resources situation, existing resources may be guarded, further limiting the quality of care provided and adding to the potential for burnout in the care provider.

Functions. The human services organization exists to promote and maintain the welfare of the public. Since society defines the functions of human service organizations, there are numerous outside controls on the operations of any one agency (Perrow, 1979). Consequently, care providers may be unclear as to who defines their responsibilities and how they are to fulfill their responsibilities. Such ambiguity and confusion about the work to be performed and lines of responsibility undermine the care provider's sense of accomplishment and may contribute to the development of burnout.

Roles. The human services organization determines the role behavior expected of care providers and the nature of interconnections among positions within the organization (Katz & Kahn, 1978). The extent to which role expectations are incongruent with the expectations and expertise of care providers results in role conflict and may contribute to the development of burnout. In addition, human service organizations may require that professional employees assume many roles within the organization, thus contributing to work overload and inability to derive a sense of satisfaction within their sphere of professional expertise and practice.

Care Recipients

The axis representing the care recipient includes individual and demographic characteristics, chronicity, acuity, and complexity of problem variables. The impact of care recipient variables as they relate to the development of burnout in care providers is neglected in the literature. However, the nature of care recipients defines the nature of services provided, and the parameters of the helping relationship define the nature of the interaction with care providers. When the demands of care recipients

tion with care providers. When the demands of care recipients exceed the capabilities of care providers or the resources of the human service organization to support the care provider, the care provider is threatened and may experience a loss of self esteem as a helping individual, thus increasing the potential for the development of burnout.

Individual behaviors. Individual behavior that might impact on the stress of the helping relationship and the utilization of organizational resources include behavioral manifestations of personality such as anger, anxiety, hostility, and despair. These characteristics challenge the competency of the care provider as a professional and as a person. While it may be possible for the care provider to cope with one recipient who displays negative feelings, the coping strategies are depleted by the cumulative affect of an entire caseload of recipients with similar negative affects.

Demographic variables. Demographic variables of care recipients that have been associated with burnout in care providers include recipient age, gender, marital and family status, education, ethnicity, and socioeconomic status. Recipient age impacts on the development of burnout in that the very young and very old require the appropriation of a greater variety of resources, and greater adaptation in the delivery of services. Each age group may evoke unique rescue fantasies on the part of the care provider, thus adding to potential energy depletion. For example, the care provider may feel an additional responsibility to help a child because of the potential for long-term impact on the child's life, and consequently, devote additional resources to the child's care to the detriment of self.

There are no studies to document the relationship between marital and family status of care recipients and burnout in care providers. However, it may be hypothesized that marital and family status represent potential supports for care recipients, thus directly impacting on the intensity of services needed and the potential resolution of the problem. In studies of blue collar workers, social support has been linked to the reduction of occupational stress and the improvement of health status (Cooper & Payne, 1980; House, 1981).

The educational level, social economic status, and ethnic background of care recipients all potentially impact on the development of burnout in care providers. The degree to which care recipients are perceived as similar or different from the care provider determines the effort required by the care provider to understand and define recipient problems and to implement acceptable and realistic solutions. Lack of education and economic resources are linked with complexity of care recipient problems and recidivism, thus further taxing the competencies and resources of the care provider and the human service organization.

Chronicity. Chronicity of care recipient problems is an influence on the helping relationship. Because chronic problems are unsolvable, the care provider may question the meaningfulness of efforts to provide services commensurate with the situation. Studies have found high burnout rates among care providers working with child abuse clients, mentally retarded clients, and chronically ill psychiatric patients (Daley, 1979; Maslach, 1982). These care recipients present problems that thwart the expectation of the care provider for resolution of the problem.

Acuity. Likewise, acuity or the immediacy and intensity of care recipient problems, is a contributing factor to burnout. The human element of the care recipient problems that are brought to care providers adds a sense of immediacy and crisis to the provision of services in human service organizations. The acuity of the problems may necessitate a decision based upon ambiguous and incomplete information. Consequently, the care provider may continuously question the quality of decisions and the appropriateness of solutions. In addition, the acuity of the situation may preclude consultation and verification processes usually available to clarify and provide support in ambiguous situations, further augmenting the sense of stress in the care provider in the situation.

Complexity. Complexity of care recipient problems or the multiproblem client places additional stresses on the care provider and the human service organization. Such problems require the expenditure of additional resources and the mobilization of interinstitutional and interagency resources. Consequently, complex problems complicate the communication and decision making structures and process, thus further stressing the delivery system and the care provider.

Dynamics of the Multidimensional Approach

The proposed approach is a representation of variables associated with the provider of care, the organization, and the recipient of care as they impact on the development of burnout. Each cell of the approach represents a subsystem of the larger system. Each cell represents the cumulative effect of three variables, one from each axis. A basic assumption of the approach is that an optimal relationship is required among variables within each cell to prevent the occurrence of burnout. For example, a cell that represents the convergence of care recipients' acuity, organizational resources, and care provider's expertise necessitates a balance between the acuity of the care recipient's problems, the resources for effective care, and the expertise of the care provider. Conversely, if either the expertise of the care provider is inadequate, or the requirements of the organization increase without adjustments in support, or the acuity of the care recipient intensifies, there is potential for the development of burnout.

IMPLICATIONS

The approach facilitates the comprehensive investigation of variables identified in the literature as associated with burnout. Placing the variables in a three dimensional matrix which includes the care recipient as well as the care provider and the organization provides the basis for theoretical formulations of burnout specific to human service organizations. such an approach enables the manipulation of specific independent variables and the measurement of the relationship between those variables.

Descriptive and experimental research is needed to further develop and validate the approach as a realistic representation of the burnout phenomenon in human services organizations. Descriptive studies designed to document the salient characteristics of each of the variables included in the approach and to determine the inclusiveness of the variables as operationalization in the approach are needed. For example, which attributes of a professional status are associated with burnout rates in care providers and in which particular organizational structures? To what extent are limitations on the dispersions of the resources of a human service organization a contributing factor in the development of burnout? Controlled studies are needed to determine relationships between the variables as the approach is applied to specific situations common to the delivery of human services. Systematic investigation of the relationships between each of the variables along one axis with each of the variables along the other axes are needed. The approach provides a structure for the generation of hypotheses. For example: The development of burnout in care providers is related to a decrease in human service resources and to an increase in complexity of care recipient's needs; the development of burnout in the care providers is related to an increase in task specificity and an increase in the chronicity of the care recipient; the intensity of burnout in care providers will decrease in relation to increase in authority while care recipient characteristics remain constant. Investigation of these and other hypotheses will contribute to an understanding of variables associated with burnout.

In addition, the approach provides a structure for assessing human service delivery situations and for predicting the potential for burnout to occur in a dysfunctional situation. Such an assessment can be made according to the interrelationship of the identified variables associated with care recipients, care providers, and human service organizations. It might be hypothesized, for example, that given projected budget restrictions and the projected turnover in care providers, the frequency of burnout will increase while care recipient characteristics remain constant.

The approach also provides a structure for the systematic identification of variables operational in a burnout situation. Thus, the approach enables the testing of intervention strategies specifically targeted toward those variables that are amenable to adjustment. In addition, the possible consequences of intervention strategies on the other salient components of the system may be predicted, an essential element when intervening in human situations. If the variables and potential relationships were identified by the model, then the effectiveness of intervention strategies could be anticipated, monitored, and evaluated.

In summary, the conceptual approach presents relationships between care providers, human service organizations, and the recipients of care in the development of burnout in the providers of human services. The multidimensionality of the approach suggests research possibilities, and suggests that burnout is a complicated phenomenon.

REFERENCES

Berglund, K. & Permelia, D. (1979). The relationship between burnout and support. Master's thesis, University of Michigan.
Berkeley Planning Associates (1977). *Project management and worker burnout: Final report*, (Vol. IX). Berkeley, CA.
Bramhall, M. & Ezell, S. How agencies can prevent burnout. *Public Welfare, 39*(3), 33-37.
Cooper, C. L. & Payne, R. (eds.). (1980). *Current concepts in occupational stress*. New York: John Wiley & Sons.
Corcoran, K. J. & Bryce, A. K. (1983). Intervention in the experience of burnout: Effects of skill development. *Journal of Social Service Research, 7*(1), 71-79.
Daley, M. R. (1979). Burnout: Smoldering problem in protective services. *Social Worker, 24*(5), 375-379.
Edelwich, J. & Brodsky, A. (1980). *Burnout: Stages of disillusionment in the helping professions*. New York: Human Sciences Press.
Freudenberger, H. J. (1975). The staff burnout syndrome in alternative institutions. *Psychotherapy: Theory, Research and Practice, 12*(1), 73-82.
Freudenberger, J. J. & Richelson, G. (1980). *Burnout: The high cost of achievement*. New York: Anchor.
Gann, M. L. (1979). The role of personality factors and job characteristics in burnout: A study of social service workers (Doctoral dissertation, University of California-Berkeley, 1979). *Dissertation Abstracts International, 34,* 07a, 80000351-3366.
Gillespie, D. F. (1981). Correlates for active and passive types of burnout. *Journal of Social Service Research, 4*(2), 1-16.
Hall, R. H. (1982). *Organizations: Structure and process*. Englewood Cliffs, NJ: Prentice-Hall.
Hasenfeld, Y. (1983). *Human service organizations*. Englewood Cliffs, NJ: Prentice-Hall.
Heckman, S. J. (1981). Effects of work setting, theoretical orientation and personality on psychotherapist burnout (Doctoral dissertation, University of California-Berkeley, 1980). *Dissertation Abstracts International, 41*(12), 8110175-466-B.
House, J. S. & Wells, J. A. (1978). Occupational stress, social support, and health. In A. McLean (ed.), *Reducing occupational stress: Proceedings of a conference*

(DHEW [N10SH] Publication No. 78-140). Washington, DC: U.S. Government Printing Office.
House, J. S. (1981). *Work stress and social support*. Reading, MA: Addison-Wesley Publishing.
Katz, D. & Kahn, R.L. (1978). *The social psychology of organizations*. 2nd ed. New York: John Wiley & Sons.
Larson, C. C., Gilbertson, D. L. & Powell, J. A. (1978). Therapist burnout: Perspectives on a critical issue. *Social Casework, 59*(6), 563-565.
Maslach, C. (1982). *Burnout: The cost of caring*. Englewood Cliffs, NJ: Prentice-Hall.
Maslach, C. & Jackson, S. E. (1981). The measurement of experienced burnout. *Journal of Occupational Behavior, 2,* 99-113.
Perlman, B. & Hartman, E. A. (1982). Burnout: Summary and future research. *Human Relations, 35*(4), 283-305.
Perrow, C. (1979). *Complex organizations*. Glenview, IL: Scott, Foresman and Co.
Pines, A. M., Aronson, E. & Kafry, D. (1981). *Burnout: From tedium to personal growth*. New York: The Free Press.
Solomon, J. R. (1979). Additional perspectives on therapist burnout. *Social Casework, 60*(6), 563-565.
Steers, R. M. (1977). Antecedents and outcomes of organizational commitment. *Administrative Science Quarterly, 22*(1), 46-56.
Sutton, R. I. & Ford, L. H. (1982). Problem-solving adequacy in hospital subunits. *Human Relations, 35*(8), 675-701.
Warshaw, A. (1979). *Managing stress*. Reading, MA: Addison-Wesley Publishing.
Weiner, M. E. (1982). *Human service management: Analysis and application*. Homewood, IL: Dorsey.

Factors Associated with Burnout in the Social Services: An Exploratory Study

Craig Winston LeCroy
Mark R. Rank

SUMMARY. Based upon a sample of 106 social workers, factors related to burnout are examined. Several variables related to the job structure within the social services emerge as potentially important determinants of burnout. These include satisfaction, autonomy, self-esteem, and discrepancy. It would appear that the source of the burnout problem is more a function of the job situation than a function of individual personality. A social service agency will obtain higher worker effectiveness and less worker exhaustion by recognizing the need for worker independence, self-esteem, acceptance, and support.

Increasing concern has been voiced regarding job-related stress among human services professionals. Social work can be seen as a job which carries a variety of inherent stresses. The nature of social work activity, the problems that social workers must confront, the limitations of knowledge and professional ability, and the structure of the social work profession all converge to produce a job with inherent stresses. Moreover, social work has historically accepted as its task the responsibility and burden of affirming and implementing moral and social values,

---

Dr. LeCroy is Assistant Professor, School of Social Work, Arizona State University, Tempe, AZ 85287 and Dr. Rank is Assistant Professor, Department of Sociology, Washington University, St. Louis, MO 63130. Requests for reprints should be addressed to Dr. LeCroy. The authors would like to acknowledge the work of the following people on this project: Judy Davidson, Mari Koeplin, Duffy Peet, Deb Ranger, Kenneth Reid, John Wise and Ruth Yarger.

© 1987 by The Haworth Press, Inc. All rights reserved.

to which society may give only contradictory or partial expression and support (Rapoport, 1960). Richan and Mendelson suggest that social work has become the "unloved Profession" (Richan & Mendelson, 1973). Indeed, the social worker's environment can be quite demanding. Larson, Gilbertson and Powell (1978) call attention to the continual responsibility of meeting the emotional needs and desires of clients that social workers must face. They point out that social workers must be ready to clarify, confront, encourage, suggest, entice, frustrate and feel for clients as the occasion demands. This kind of emotional investment and its effects have been widely discussed in the literature (Burton, 1975; English, 1976; Gillespie, 1980; Pines & Maslach, 1978). However, research on this important topic has not been forthcoming (Gillespie, 1983).

The depth and complexity of factors contributing to burnout is great. How these variables are associated with burnout will vary with the individual and the organization. This research examines the influence of psychological, demographic, and occupational background variables upon burnout. Of particular interest is the extent to which the following psychological constructs are related to burnout: job satisfaction, professional self-esteem, work autonomy, discrepancy, ability to cope, and assertiveness. These constructs are discussed below.

REVIEW OF THE LITERATURE

Job Satisfaction

The relationship between burnout and job satisfaction has received considerable attention (Harrison, 1980; Jayaratne & Chess, 1983, 1984). Harrison (1980) uses the concept of job satisfaction and assumes it is closely related to the concept of burnout. However, the extent to which these concepts are overlapping has not received much study. Jayaratne and Chess (1983) did investigate the relationship between job satisfaction and two indices of burnout, depersonalization and emotional exhaustion. While overlap was evident, the authors note that the two concepts are not identical. In order to continue to examine this relationship, the analysis includes job satisfaction as a predictor of burnout. It is hypothesized that job satisfaction will be negatively related to burnout.

Professional Self-Esteem and Work Autonomy

Kermish and Kushin (1969) examined the reasons for high turnover in a public welfare setting and found that job dissatisfaction and turnover were associated with the workers' belief that they were unable to help their clients, were not given proper respect, and could not be creative and use their own initiative. Dorman (1971) presents findings that suggest the more bureaucratic the organization, the lower the level of professionalism. Additionally, Dorman indicates bureaucratic agencies produce minimal feelings of autonomy by workers. Furthermore, Clearfield (1977) has found that social workers with a positive professional image develop a sense of identity with their work and are happier than those who are deprived of professional self-esteem.

It is hypothesized that positive professional self-esteem will be negatively correlated with burnout. Professional self-esteem is seen as a subjective evaluation regarding the prestige of the social worker's job, the worth of the profession and its opportunities for personal growth, self-fulfillment, and service to other people provided by the profession (Kim, Boo & Wheeler, 1978). Additionally, it is hypothesized that an increase in work autonomy, like professional self-esteem, will be negatively associated with burnout.

Discrepancy

Work autonomy and professional self-esteem are often measured by examining "how much is there" items and "how much there should be" items across several facets. This allows for measuring the worker's present level of attainment and that worker's aspirations (Dehlinger & Perlman, 1978). This technique of discrepancy measurement gives an indication of perceived deficiency in need fulfillment. It is hypothesized that increases in discrepancy will be positively correlated with burnout.

Ability to Cope

A person's ability to cope is likely to affect burnout. Interpersonal support systems can be seen as protective buffers against work stresses and reduce the amount of tedium a person experiences (Pines & Kafry, 1978). Recent findings (Maslach & Pines, 1977; Pines & Kafry, 1978; Scholom & Perlman, 1979) suggest that a positive social milieu may provide this buffer to significantly reduce job stress. Austin et al. (1977) found that eighty percent of the social workers interviewed found it helpful to share job-related concerns with their spouse or roommate when under pressure. From this, an index was devised to measure a person's ability to cope.

Assertiveness

Larson, Gilbertson and Powell (1978) discuss how not setting limits can lead a social worker to burnout. "By failing to say 'no,' within reason, to the demands of their communities and governing boards, and by failing to educate the communities to accept their limits, they, in turn, set the stage for their own incompetence and burnout" (p. 564). This suggests the importance of examining whether or not assertiveness, as a personality construct, has any effect on the burnout indices.

METHOD

Sampling

A nonrandom sample was identified for use in the present study. A list of social service agencies was generated in two midwestern towns in two different states. From this list phone calls were made to identify social workers who were employed at the agencies. The workers were then contacted and asked to participate in an interview. Because the communities where this research was conducted were relatively small it was not possible to randomly sample from a larger universe of social service agencies. Consequently, the sample is one of convenience. The personal contacts with the social workers allowed for an open interview format as well as the administration of a questionnaire. This method was chosen over mailed questionnaires so that a larger sample would be obtained over what could be expected if the subjects were asked to complete and mail questionnaires on their own recognizance. All subjects who agreed to be interviewed completed the questionnaire. Only six social workers refused to be interviewed for the study. The entire sample was 106 respondents.

Measurement

The first section of the questionnaire consisted of 14 demographic and occupational background questions including age, sex, education, and nature of the social service job. The second section included 25 questions of the Maslach Burnout Inventory. The third section consisted of 47 questions covering factors which were hypothesized to contribute to burnout. These factors included job satisfaction and autonomy, professional self-esteem, discrepancy, coping mechanisms, and personal assertiveness.

In order to establish the degree of burnout experienced by an individual subject, the Maslach Burnout Inventory, consisting of 25 questions measured on a seven point scale, was used in its complete form. The inventory measures four dimensions of burnout, including emotional exhaustion, negative cynical attitudes toward recipients (depersonalization), negative evaluation of the subject's own strengths and accomplishments in working with others (reduced personal accomplishment), and the subject's sense of closeness to clients. Reliability data for the subscales ranged from .71 to .90 (see Maslach & Jackson, 1981).

A modified version of Brayfield and Rothe's (1951) scale was adopted for use as the job satisfaction index. It included questions on job satisfaction, interest, enjoyment, disappointment, boredom and satisfaction with the agency. Feelings of dissatisfaction and unpleasantness were also covered. All items were scaled as strongly agree to strongly disagree. The authors report a reliability estimate of .87 for the scale.

The job autonomy and professional self-esteem indices were based on the work of Porter and Lawler (1968) as adopted by Kim, Boo and Wheeler (1978). Job autonomy was measured by such questions as the amount of individual authority connected with one's position, one's opportunity for determining methods and procedures, one's opportunity for independent thought and action, and one's opportunity for participation in the setting of goals. These were measured, as perceived by the subject, on a seven-point scale of "minimal" to "maximum." Information on the reliability of these instruments was unavailable.

Professional self-esteem was measured on the same seven-point scale. Questions included the opportunity in one's position to give help to other people; the prestige of one's position, both within and outside the agency; feelings of security, worthwhile accomplishment, self-fulfillment and self-esteem in one's position; and one's opportunity for personal growth and development.

The professional self-esteem and work autonomy items were each followed by the question, "How much should there be?" This was then subtracted from the initial response, resulting in our measurement of discrepancy.

Coping mechanisms included both job-oriented and personal supports. This area was measured on a four-point scale with most questions rated from "never" to "usually." Job-oriented questions included the gaining of emotional support from a supervisor, involvement in career-related organizations and agency support groups, ability to share feelings with co-workers and days off for mental health. Non-work related supports that were measured included the presence of emotional strength within family, time spent with a spouse or significant other, a philosophical or religious belief, planned social activities with non-agency friends, physical exercise, recreational activities, and personal time for oneself. This measure was developed for the present research.

The assertiveness scale was adapted and modified from the work of Gambrill and Richey (1975). Assertiveness was measured on a point scale by questions which examined personal characteristics indicating assertive behavior. Questions included the frequency an individual would ask a favor, express differing opinions, resist pressure, and interrupt a talkative person.

RESULTS

Table 1 presents a general picture of the sample. Three portions of this table warrant discussion. First, almost half of the respondents were between the ages of 20 and 30 years old, with another 31 percent between 31 to 40 years of age. Together, this comprises 80 percent of the sample who are 40 years of age or younger.

The other portions of Table 1 needing further elaboration are the number of years in full-time employment in the field of social work. In response to the full-time employment question, 60 percent of the sample responded that they had been in the field for six years or less. It is interesting to compare this with the responses from the numbers of years in current position question. On this question, 91 percent of the sample stated that they had been in their current position six years or less. This includes 69 percent of the sample who answered the question with zero to three years in their current position. This may reflect the amount of job turnover within the profession with individuals changing from one agency to another or a promotional role change.

Demographic and Occupational Background Characteristics

The indicators of burnout varied only slightly across the demographic and occupational background variables. For example, marital status, ethnic background, educational level, and job title did not vary by major variable. Particularly interesting are the results on job title which showed a lack of difference between practitioner, supervisor and administrator on emotional exhaustion.

On the negative feelings index, gender was significant, $F(1,106) = 10.11$, $p < .002$ with females scoring much lower on negative feelings toward recipients than males. Additionally, females scored significantly lower on the closeness to the recipients index when compared with males, $F(1,106) = 9.70$, $p <$

TABLE 1. Demographic and Occupational Background Characteristics of Surveyed Respondents

Demographic Characteristics	Percentage	Occupational Background Characteristics	Percentage
Age		**Job Title**	
20-30	49	Practitioner	65
21-40	31	Supervisor	8
41-50	11	Administrator	12
51-60	8	Other	15
61-over	1	Total	100%
Total	100%		
		Salary	
Sex		Below $10,000	6
Female	61	$10,000-$15,000	43
Male	39	$16,000-$20,000	37
Total	100%	$21,000-$25,000	9
		$26,000-above	5
Marital Status		Total	100%
Single	23	**Number of Years in Current Position**	
Married	67		
Divorced	9		
Other	1	0-3	69
Total	100%	4-6	22
		7-9	6
Race or Ethnic Background		10-12	1
		13-15	1
Black	16	16-more	1
White	79	Total	100%
American Indian	2		
Hispanic	2	**Number of Years in Full-Time Employment in Field of Social Work**	
Other	1		
Total	100%		
		0-3	27
Educational Level		4-6	33
		7-9	14
Ph.D.	4	10-12	9
M.S.W.	50	13-15	4
B.A. or B.S.	46	16-18	5
		19-21	2
Total	100%	22-more	6
		Total	100%

.002. Gender differences did not emerge on the measures of emotional exhaustion or reduced personal accomplishment.

An interesting finding is that salary range had a significant effect on the emotional exhaustion index, $F(4,102) = 3.5$, $p < .01$. Emotional exhaustion tends to decrease as salary increases. This is particularly true for workers who made less than $20,000 compared to workers in the $26,000 and above salary range.

Unexpectedly, the number of years in current position did not produce significant results on most of the predicted variables.

There was, however, one significant difference in the feelings of closeness to recipients index, $F(4,102) = 3.53$, $p < .01$, showing an association between less time spent in one's current position and the closer one felt to recipients.

Contrary to expectation, emotional exhaustion, depersonalization, and closeness to recipients did not increase with the number of hours spent in direct client contact or time spent working overtime hours.

Table 2 shows the means, standard deviations and numbers for each concentration in the social work field on the emotional exhaustion index. Child abuse workers had the highest mean on emotional exhaustion index. Child abuse, as an area of concentration, was considerably higher on emotional exhaustion than the other areas. Child abuse workers also had high means compared with the other concentrations on the indexes of negative feelings and closeness to recipients. The latter finding tends to support Maslach's theory that an important factor associated with burnout is the closeness felt toward clients.

Table 3 presents the mean raw score, the range of possible scores, and the standard deviations across all major variables. Emotional exhaustion had a mean of 50.86 with a large standard deviation indicating that many social workers feel moderate to strong stress and exhaustion from working at their job. In terms of percentage, 10 percent of the sample indicated they felt burned out from their work either daily or a few times a week; 32 percent felt this way either weekly or a few times a month. When an-

TABLE 2. Area of Concentration by Emotional Exhaustion

Area of Concentration	Mean	Standard deviation	Size
Child Abuse	70.45	15.83	11
Child Welfare	57.18	23.71	16
Mental Health--Outpatient	43.84	18.00	25
Mental Health--Institutional	44.30	17.91	10
Service to Families	51.00	24.10	15

TABLE 3. Mean Scores and Standard Deviations of Burnout Factors

Variable	Range	Mean	Standard deviation
Emotional Exhaustion	0-90	50.86	21.37
Depersonalization	0-75	36.18	12.04
Reduced Personal Accomplishment	0-75	16.70	10.87
Closeness to Recipients	0-45	15.26	6.37

swering how strongly this was felt, 59 percent of the workers responded from moderate to very strong.

Correlational Analysis

Table 4 presents the product-moment correlations between the factors of burnout and the psychological dimensions mentioned earlier. These results will be discussed separately, looking at each major variable in detail.

Job satisfaction. As hypothesized, job satisfaction is negatively correlated with burnout. The correlations are significant

TABLE 4. Product-Moment Correlations Between Psychological Constructs and Factors of Burnout

Burnout Factors	Psychological Constructs							
	X^1	X^2	X^3	X^4	X^5	X^6	X^7	X^8
Emotional Exhaustion	-.65**	-.47**	-.30**	.33**	.42**	.41**	-.34**	-.18
Depersonalization	-.27**	-.17	-.21*	.27**	.29**	.32**	-.12	.08
Reduced Personal Accomplishment	-.50**	-.59**	-.35**	.22	.37**	.33**	-.37	-.10
Closeness to Recipients	-.13	-.14	-.15	-.19	.26	.26**	.06	-.02

N = 106

*significant at the .05 level
**significant at the .01 level

Key: X_1 = Job Satisfaction
X_2 = Professional Self-Esteem
X_3 = Job Autonomy
X_4 = Work Autonomy Discrepancy
X_5 = Self-Esteem Discrepancy
X_7 = Combined Discrepancy ($X^4 + X^5$)
X_8 = Coping Ability
X_6 = Assertiveness

for emotional exhaustion, negative feelings, and negative job evaluation. Hence, the more satisfied an individual feels in his or her job setting, the less likely s/he is to experience burnout.

Professional self-esteem and work autonomy. The correlational results (not presented here) show job autonomy to be closely related to professional self-esteem ($r = .76$, $p < .01$), indicating that work autonomy and professional self-esteem seem to be interrelated. Positive professional self-esteem is negatively related to all factors of burnout, as hypothesized. There is a significant negative correlation with both emotional exhaustion ($r = -.47$, $p < .01$) and reduced personal accomplishment ($r = -.59$, $p < .01$).

Similarly, an increase in job autonomy, like professional self-esteem, is negatively correlated to all factors of burnout, as predicted. The product-moment correlations produced significant results with emotional exhaustion ($r = -.30$, $p < .01$), depersonalization ($r = -.21$, $p < .05$), and reduced personal accomplishment ($r = -.35$, $p < .01$).

Workers who report greater job autonomy and professional self-esteem are likely to have greater job competency. This finding is similar to results reported by Kermish and Kushin (1969) who found that job dissatisfaction and turnover was associated with the workers' inability to help clients, lack of respect and limited ability to be creative and use their own initiative.

These results also support Clearfield's (1977) contention that social workers with a positive professional image develop a sense of identity with their work and are happier than those deprived of professional self-esteem. Persons exhibiting low professional self-esteem may over-compensate for their negative feelings by over-involvement with clients or have unrealistic goals about their effectiveness on the job. These studies suggest that several factors cluster together forming an interrelated association between persons with high professional self-esteem, work autonomy, job competence, job satisfaction and coping mechanisms which all interact to decrease emotional exhaustion and other factors of burnout.

Discrepancy. In contrast to the above, it was hypothesized that increases in discrepancy would be positively associated with the factors of burnout. As expected, a worker experiencing more discrepancy is associated with indications of burnout. For example, looking at combined discrepancy, the data show fairly strong positive correlations with emotional exhaustion (r = .41, p < .01), negative feelings (r = .32, p < .01), negative job evaluation (r = .33, p < .01), and closeness to recipients (r = .26, p < .01).

Workers who are experiencing a perceived deficiency in need fulfillment may be less satisfied with their jobs and may be more likely to burnout. Maslach (1976) refers to a loss of balanced perspective and suggests that this may be a beginning symptom of burnout. Cherniss, Egnatios and Wacker (1976) expand on this and claim that it is the conflict between the service ideal and bureaucratic demands that puts undue stress on the worker. The discrepancy measure may be an indication of this conflict as well as the professional mystique which leads to unrealistic expectations and disillusionment.

Ability to cope. The major hypothesis with regard to coping mechanisms was that the more coping mechanisms a person used, the less likely he or she would experience burnout. This hypothesis was supported by the negative correlation found between coping mechanisms and emotional exhaustion (r = −.34, p < .01) as well as negative job evaluation (r = −.37, p < .01). Negative feelings correlated in the predicted direction with coping mechanisms but was not significant.

When on the job coping mechanisms were separated from the personal coping mechanisms, on the job factors had greater negative associations with burnout than personal coping mechanisms. Social workers are interactors and communicators, and involvement and support from supervisor, co-worker and professional colleague is an important factor in preserving effective interaction with clients. These results suggest the need for social workers to balance their giving to clients with effective positive supports, both within and outside the work environment. These results concur with the finding of Maslach and Pines (1977) that staff meetings perceived as having supportive value are closely related to better working conditions. More recently, Gillespie and Cohen (1984) found that workers' dissatisfaction with their supervisors was one of the major causes of burnout in child protective services.

Assertiveness. Assertiveness was expected to help reduce burnout. While assertiveness and both emotional exhaustion and negative job evaluation did correlate in the predicted direction, neither was statistically significant. On the other hand, assertiveness and negative feelings are positively related.

The lack of support on the assertiveness measure requires some explanation. It may be that the assertiveness index was neither broad enough nor finely demarcated enough to detect the differences between non-assertive, assertive, and aggressive behavior. In addition, assertiveness had the smallest standard deviation, of the measures used, indicating little variance on the assertiveness index. On the other hand, it may be that assertiveness is simply not an important factor in predicting burnout.

Multiple Regression Analysis

Table 5 presents additional analysis based on multiple regression equations. The four burnout factors were used as criterion variables and they were regressed on the remaining major variables. By doing so, the independent importance of the psychological constructs upon burnout can be assessed.

In each regression equation, one or two variables emerged as significant. Emotional exhaustion had one significant predictor, job satisfaction. Self-esteem discrepancy was significant in predicting depersonalization, reduced personal accomplishment, and closeness to recipients. Lastly, professional self-esteem was negatively related to poor job evaluation.

By taking the combined burnout factors together, discrepancy emerges as the best independent predictor. Professional self-esteem discrepancy explains the most in terms of the various factors which are used to define the concept of burnout. Discrepancy may represent the workers' degree of conflict between what their ideal is and what they are able to accomplish within the constraints of their jobs. Differing expectations frequently led to difficulties in relationships, jobs, and feelings of life satisfaction. Given these relationships, the implication is for more effort to be expended in reducing the conflict between the ideal and the realistic aspects of social work. As Cherniss et al. (1976) suggest, problems with the "professional mystique" need to be addressed.

TABLE 5. Multiple Regression Equations for Factors of Burnout

Independent Variables	Burnout Factors			
	Emotional Exhaustion	Depersonal- ization	Reduced Personal Accomplishment	Closeness to Recipients
Job Satisfaction	-.62***	-.24	-.19	-.03
Professional Self-Esteem	-.09	.37	-.84***	.17
Job Autonomy	.12	-.13	.22	-.07
Self-Esteem Discrepancy	-.01	.35*	.31**	.41**
Coping Ability	-.05	-.01	-.09	.18
Assertiveness	-.05	.11	.07	-.01
R^2	.43	.14	.43	.11
Adjusted R^2	.40	.09	.40	.05

N = 106
*significant at the .05 level
**significant at the .01 level
***significant at the .001 level

CONCLUSION

The results of this exploratory study reinforce some of the material that has previously been written on burnout and also indicates new directions to be considered. From the demographic data, respondent's gender had a direct relationship with emotional exhaustion and closeness to recipients. Males scored significantly lower on the emotional exhaustion factor and higher on the closeness to recipients factor. It may be that men and women experience these factors in completely different ways. The implication is that we need to consider different prescriptions in devising programs and managing organizations which help social workers resist becoming burned out.

The correlational and multiple regression results turned up several factors which contribute to worker burnout. In some respects the data support Maslach's (1978) contention that the source of the burnout problem is more a function of the job situation than a function of individual personality. In fact, the personality construct—assertiveness—that was hypothesized to predict burnout proved to be insignificant. Factors related to the job situation showed several relationships with the burnout indices. Professional self-esteem, work autonomy, discrepancy, and salary all resulted in significant zero order correlations with the burnout factors. The regression analysis revealed discrepancy as a contributing factor in predicting the three criterion variables: negative feelings, negative job evaluation, and closeness to recipients.

Several of the hypotheses were not supported. Particularly, job performance variables were found to show no significant relationships to burnout. These variables included direct client contact, overtime, the number of years in the field, and the number of years in current position.

This study suggests the importance of several factors related to the job structure within the social services as potentially important determinants of burnout. These include satisfaction, autonomy, self-esteem, and discrepancy. Also germane is the finding that certain areas of concentration produce higher levels of burnout across several of the indices. Much of the research in the burnout area has dealt with child protective services and these results confirm the necessity of continued investigations which examine burnout in this field of social work practice.

It is important to point out that a particular causal sequence has been presented in this paper, that certain factors lead to individuals experiencing burnout symptoms. However, while the data make these events appear logical, they do not demonstrate it. It would be plausible, for example, to argue that individuals experience burnout and as a consequence develop lower professional self-esteem. Still, the approach presented in this discussion does appear reasonable given the current knowledge about burnout, while helping to explain how burnout may come about.

In conclusion, these results point to the importance of having a better understanding of job requirements and expectations for human service workers. Indeed, the neglect of such workers' needs may have severe effects on the individual and the organization. A social service agency will obtain higher worker effectiveness and less worker exhaustion by recognizing the need for worker independence, self-esteem, acceptance, and support.

REFERENCES

Austin, M., Babcock, N., Eddy, D., Flagler, C., Ford, D., McNally, T., Thompson, M., VanderBerg, C. & Reid, K. (1977). An exploratory study of the burnout syndrome in the social work profession. Kalamazoo, MI: Western Michigan University. School of Social Work, Field Studies in Research and Practice.

Brayfield, A. H. & Rothe, H. F. (1951). An index of job satisfaction. *Journal of Applied Psychology, 35,* 307-311.

Burton, A. (1975). Therapist satisfaction. *American Journal of Psychoanalysis, 35,* 115-122.

Cherniss, C., Egnatios, E. S. & Wacker, S. (1976). Job stress and career development in new public professionals. *Professional Psychology, 7,* 428-436.

Clearfield, S. M. (1977). Professional self-image of the social worker: Implications for social work education. *Journal of Education for Social Work, 13,* 23-30.

Dehlinger, J. & Perlman, B. (1978). Job satisfaction in mental health agencies. *Administration in Mental Health, 5,* 120-139.

Dorman, P. M. (1971). Professionalism and bureaucracy in public welfare: A study of selected agencies in the intermountain regions. Salt Lake City: University of Utah, unpublished doctoral dissertation.

English, S. O. (1976). The emotional stress of psychotherapeutic practice. *American Academy of Psychoanalysis, 4,* 119-123.

Gambrill, E. D. & Richey, C. A. (1975). An assertion inventory for use in assessment and research. *Behavior Therapy, 6,* 550-561.

Gillespie, D. F. (1980). Correlates for active and passive types of burnout. *Journal of Social Service Research, 4,* 1-16.

Gillespie, D. F. & Cohen, S. E. (1984). Causes of worker burnout. *Child and Youth Services, 6,* 115-124.

Harrison, W. D. (1980). Role strain and burnout in child-protective service workers. *Social Service Review, 54,* 31-44.

Jayaratne, S. & Chess, W. A. (1983). *Stress and burnout in the human service professions.* New York: Pergamon.

Jayaratne, S. & Chess, W. A. (1984). Job satisfaction, burnout, and turn-over: A national study. *Social Work, 29,* 448-453.

Kermish, I. & Kushin, F. (1969). Why high turnover? Social work staff losses in a county welfare agency. *Public Welfare, 27,* 134-139.

Kim, D. I., Boo, S. L. & Wheeler, A. (1978). Professional competency, autonomy and job satisfaction among social workers in an Appalachian rural area. Paper presented at the National Institute on Social Work in Rural Areas, Morgantown, WV, August 7-10, 1978.

Larson, C. C., Gilbertson, D. L. & Powell, J. A. (1978). Therapist burnout: Perspectives on a critical issue. *Social Casework, 59,* 563-565.

Maslach, C. (1976). Burned-out. *Human Behavior, 5,* 17-22.

Maslach, C. (1978). Job burnout: How people cope. *Public Welfare, 36,* 56-58.

Maslach, C. & Jackson, S. E. (1979). Burned-out cops and their families. *Psychology Today, 12,* 58-62.

Maslach, C. & Jackson, S. E. (1981). The measurement of experienced burnout. *Journal of Occupational Behavior, 2,* 99-113.

Maslach, C. & Pines, A. (1977). The burnout syndrome in the day care setting. *Child Care Quarterly, 6*, 100-113.

Pines, A. & Kafry, D. (1978). Occupational tedium in the social services. *Social Work, 23*, 499-506.

Pines, A. & Maslach, C. (1978). Characteristics of staff burnout in mental health settings. *Hospital and Community Psychiatry, 29*, 233-237.

Porter, L. W. & Lawler, E. E., III (1968). *Managerial attitudes and performance.* Homewood, IL: Irwin.

Rapoport, L. (1960). In defense of social work: An examination of stress in the profession. *Social Service Review, 34*, 62-74.

Richan, W. C. & Mendelson, A. P. (1973). *Social work: The unloved profession.* New York: New Viewpoints.

Scholom, A. & Perlman, B. (1979). Who cares for the care givers. *Administration in Mental Health, 3*, 206-216.

Gender Differences in Work Stress Among Clinical Social Workers

David P. Himle
Srinika D. Jayaratne
Wayne A. Chess

SUMMARY. Since no consistent pattern of gender differences in the measurement of burnout and work stress has been reported in the literature, this study presents further data illustrating the effect of various work-related stress variables upon burnout and selected psychological strains related to gender differences. The data were received from a national sample of 617 clinical social workers. The results indicate gender differences in the prediction of burnout and psychological strains utilizing multiple regression analyses. The nature of these differences and the implications of these findings for the reduction of work stress are discussed.

A few studies examining gender differences in burnout and work stress have been reported in the literature. Such gender differences have been reported in studies utilizing the Maslach Burnout Inventory (MBI) scales (Maslach & Jackson, 1981, 1985; Jayaratne, Tripodi & Chess, 1983). These studies report that females score significantly higher than males on the MBI emotional exhaustion subscale, but present mixed results on the MBI depersonalization and personal accomplishment subscales. On the other hand, a number of studies have reported no significant gender differences on various MBI scales and on the Burnout/Alienation scale developed by Berkeley Planning Associates

---

Drs. Himle and Jayaratne are Associate Professors at the School of Social Work, the University of Michigan, Ann Arbor, MI, 48109. Dr. Chess is Professor at the School of Social Work, University of Oklahoma, Norman, OK. Requests for reprints may be addressed to Dr. D. Himle. This paper was presented at the World Congress of Behavior Therapy, Washington, DC, 1983 (December 8-11).

(Maslach & Jackson, 1985; Jayaratne, Tripodi & Chess, 1983; Berkeley Planning Associates, 1977; Shinn, Rosario, March & Chesnut, 1981; Justice, Gold & Klein, 1981). Since no consistent pattern of gender differences in the measurement of burnout has been reported in this literature, it is the purpose of this study to examine the effect of selected job-related stress variables as predictors of burnout and selected psychological strains. This direction of research is also important since burnout has been shown to be a multifaceted concept. It has been operationally defined as a multifaceted psychological construct (Morrow, 1981), a work process phenomenon (Freudenberger, 1977), a general experience of exhaustion (Pines, Aronson & Kafry, 1981), occupational stress (Justice, Gold & Klein, 1981), and a maladaptive response to stressful situations (Maslach, 1976) and tedium (Pines & Kafry, 1978). Therefore it is our purpose to examine gender differences in work stressors as predictors of both burnout and selected psychological strains, because of this complexity. It is acknowledged that these psychological strains may be associated with what is labeled burnout, but the separate examination of these variables may result in a broader explanation of work stress than the more specific concept of burnout alone, and thus provide more useful information for the amelioration of job dissatisfaction.

THE SAMPLE

A national sample of social workers was randomly drawn from the membership list of the National Association of Social Workers. Social workers were selected as the sample since few studies have been undertaken to examine this population, and this occupation has been described as especially susceptible to the effects of burnout (Rapoport, 1960; Barrett & McKelvy, 1980; Littner, 1974; Harrison, 1980). Eleven hundred seventy four (1174) respondents were mailed a ten-page questionnaire. Eight hundred fifty-three (853) questionnaires were returned, a response rate of 70.6%. From these respondents a sample of 617 master's degree workers engaged in clinical practice were selected for this study.

The respondents were mostly female (69.4%) and predominantly white (males, 93.7%; females 88.1%). Significantly more males (78.0%) than females (58.0%) were married ($x^2 = 21.22$, df 1, p < .001). In terms of work characteristics, 48.7% of males and 57.5% of females received their MSW degrees after 1971, and 56.1% of males and 49.1% of females have been in their present social work positions for more than three years. Fifty-one and nine-tenths (51.9) percent males and 51.8% of females worked in psychiatric settings, 9.5% of males and 12.5% of females in family services agencies, 7.4% of males and 8.9% of females in private practice, 10.6% of males and 8.0% of females in school settings, and 20.6% of males and 18.8% of females in a variety of other settings. No significant differences by gender were found in these work characteristics. Significant differences by gender were found in income levels for social work positions. Seven and four-tenths (7.4) percent of males and 28.3% of females reported income less than $15,000, 58.7% of males and 59.8% of females reported income greater than $15,000 but less than $25,000, 33.9% of males and 11.9% of females reported income greater than $25,000 ($x^2 = 59.9$, df 2, p < .001).

STUDY VARIABLES

As the dependent variables for this study, we have employed three measures of psychological strain which have been used extensively in work stress research, and are considered to be generally valid and reliable (Caplan, Cobb, French, Van Harrison & Pinneau, 1975; Quinn & Staines, 1978). These measures are described as follows:

1. *Anxiety* — this index consists of 4 items with a range from 4 (never or little of the time) to 16 (most of the time). An item example is, "When you think about yourself and your job these days, how much of the time do you feel nervous?"
2. *Depression* — this index consists of 6 items with a range from 4 (never or little of the time) to 24 (most of the time). An item example is, "When you think about yourself and your job these days, how much of the time do you feel depressed?"

3. *Irritability* — this index consists of 2 items with a range from 2 (never or little of the time) to 8 (most of the time). An item example is. "When you think about yourself and your job these days, how much of the time do you feel irritated?"

In addition we used a number of measures related to the concept of burnout. The measures are from the Maslach Burnout Inventory (Maslach & Jackson, 1981). This widely used inventory is composed of three subscales which we utilized:

1. *Emotional Exhaustion subscale* — this index consists of one item, "I feel burned-out from my work." We decided to use this single item rather than the nine item scale, because this item had a factor loading of .81 with the total scale (Maslach & Jackson, 1981). The response to the item has a range from 1 (strongly disagree) to 7 (strongly agree).
2. *Depersonalization subscale* — this index consists of five items with a range from 5 (strongly disagree) to 35 (strongly agree). An item example is, "I feel I treat some recipients as if they were impersonal objects."
3. *Personal Accomplishment subscale* — this index consists of eight items with a range from 8 (strongly disagree) to 56 (strongly agree). An item example is "I feel I am positively influencing people's lives."

As independent or predictor variables we have used the following eleven measures related to the worker's evaluation of the job. These variables are perceptual measures: indices which measure how an individual views his/her job. They are not indicators of the absolute job situation context. We have used measures of different facets of work such as workload, client contact time, job comfort, and worker support. We have also used measures which assess the worker's general reaction to the job without reference to any specific job facets, such as "How likely is it that you will make a genuine effort to seek a new job next year?" This dual approach has been suggested by Quinn and Staines (1978). The following measures were used, and the sources are indicated:

1. *Emotional Support of Supervisor* — This index consists of 4 items with a range from 4 (very true) to 16 (not at all true). An item example is, "How true is it that this supervisor is warm and friendly when you are troubled about something?" (Caplan, Cobb, French, Van Harrison & Pinneau, 1975)
2. *Emotional Support of Co-workers* — This index consists of 4 items with a range from 4 (very true) to 16 (not at all true). An item example is, "How true is it that co-workers show approval when you do something well?" (Caplan, Cobb, French, Van Harrison & Pinneau, 1975)
3. *Direct Contact with Clients* — This index consists of 1 item indicating the percentage of time spent in direct contact with clients.
4. *Role Ambiguity* — This index consists of 4 items and has a score range from 4 (very often) to 20 (rarely). An item example is, "How often are you clear on what your job responsibilities are?" (Rizzo, House & Lirtzman, 1970)
5. *Role Conflict* — This index consists of 4 items and has a score range from 4 (very true) to 16 (not at all true). An item example is, "To satisfy some people on my job, I have to upset others." (Rizzo, House & Lirtzman, 1970)
6. *Work Load* — This index consists of 4 items and has a score range from 4 (very often) to 20 (rarely). An item example is, "How often does your work leave you with little time to get things done?" (Caplan, Cobb, French, Van Harrison & Pinneau, 1975)
7. *Intent to Quit* — This index consists of a single item, "How likely is it that you will make a genuine effort to seek a new job next year?" The item has a score range from 1 (very likely) to 3 (not at all likely).
8. *Sex Discrimination* — This index consists of a single item, "Do you feel in any way discriminated against on your job because of sex?" This item has a score range of 1 (feel this way frequently) to 3 (never feel this way).
9. *Job Comfort* — This index consists of 7 items with a score range of 7 (very true) to 28 (not at all true). An item example is, "The physical surroundings are pleasant." (Quinn & Sheppard, 1974)

10. *Financial Rewards* – This index consists of 3 items and has a score range from 3 (very true) to 12 (not at all true). An item example is, "The pay is good." (Quinn & Staines, 1978)
11. *Challenge* – This index consists of 6 items and has a score range from 6 (very true) to 24 (not at all true). An item example is, "On this job I am given a chance to do the things I like best." (Quinn & Sheppard, 1974)

These predictor variables measured by the indices mentioned above have been utilized by a variety of researchers in numerous settings. For example, Maslach and Pines (1977) have shown that the number of clients served is positively associated with burnout. Pines and Kafry (1978) state that women are more likely to utilize existing support systems than men in dealing with burnout. Maslach and Jackson (1981) report that those who are burned out say that they plan to leave their jobs within a year. Harrison (1980) reports that the existence of role conflict and ambiguity contributes to work stress. Maslach (1982) also has reported that a lack of supervisor support contributes to work stress. Sutton (1982) has shown that females receive fewer financial rewards than males in professions such as social work. Jayaratne and Chess (1983) have reported that lack of job challenge contributes to depersonalization. Therefore, we believe that predictor variables employed in this study are highly relevant to the issue of burnout and work stress.

RESULTS

Table 1 presents the mean scores, standard deviations and t-values for the predictor variables by gender. Four significant gender differences in work experience are evident in four areas: direct client contact (females higher than males), role ambiguity (females more frequent than males), sex discrimination (females more than males), and financial rewards (males more satisfied than females).

Table 2 presents the mean scores, standard deviations and t-

Table 1
Descriptive Statistics of Predictor Variables by Gender[1]

Variable	N	Mean	SD	T-Value
Supervisor Support				
Males	149	7.83	3.62	-.11
Females	343	7.88	3.67	
Co-Worker Support				
Males	152	7.15	2.61	1.66
Females	350	6.69	2.91	
Direct Client Contact				
Males	163	36.55	21.51	-3.84*
Females	364	44.53	22.19	
Role Ambiguity				
Males	170	8.09	3.12	2.53*
Females	386	7.42	2.72	
Role Conflict				
Males	168	9.40	3.01	.45
Females	371	9.27	3.03	
Work Load				
Males	171	8.50	3.10	1.67
Females	385	8.00	3.25	
Intent to Quit				
Males	175	2.41	.79	1.01
Females	384	2.34	.79	
Sex Discrimination				
Males	171	2.88	.36	7.67*
Females	374	2.46	.67	
Job Comfort				
Males	166	15.07	3.74	-1.32
Females	375	15.57	4.13	
Financial Rewards				
Males	168	5.94	1.97	2.80*
Females	376	6.51	2.28	
Challenge				
Males	168	10.32	3.10	.59
Females	370	10.14	3.26	

[1] Different N's reflect missing data.
* $p < .01$

values for the dependent variables. No significant differences by gender were found.

An analysis of the correlation coefficients between the eleven predictor variables by gender, showed that for males only two

Table 2
Descriptive Statistics of Dependent Variables by Gender[1]

Variable	N	Mean	SD	T-Value	
Anxiety					
Males	180	7.42	1.29	1.13	NS
Females	408	7.29	1.24		
Depression					
Males	180	12.41	1.84	-.24	NS
Females	404	12.44	1.62		
Irritability					
Males	183	3.78	1.08	.94	NS
Females	416	3.68	1.13		
Emotional Exhaustion					
Males	189	3.30	1.94	.94	NS
Females	428	3.14	1.90		
Depersonalization					
Males	182	11.52	5.20	1.56	NS
Females	422	10.80	5.09		
Personal Accomplishment					
Males	183	39.96	5.08	1.29	NS
Females	415	39.33	5.63		

[1] Different N's reflect missing data.

coefficients exceeded .49, and for females only two coefficients exceeded .49, indicating minimal multicollinearity (Cohen & Cohen, 1975).

In order to determine the relative effects of the various job related predictors of psychological strain, we conducted a standardized multiple regression analysis for each dependent variable. The resulting beta weights, and their F tests are presented in Table 3 for male and female workers.

There were no significant predictors of anxiety for males or females among the work stress variables. Furthermore, the total variance explained is minimal in both instances.

The best predictor of depression for both males and females was sex discrimination on the job, which was associated with increased depression. A decreased likelihood to quit was associated with decreased depression for females. The best predictor of depression for males was the percentage of time in direct contact

Table 3

Job Facets as Predictors: Multiple Regression Analysis on Psychological Strains

Predictors	Anxiety				Depression				Irritation			
	Males		Females		Males		Females		Males		Females	
	Beta	F Ratio	Beta	F Ratio	Beta	F Ratio	Beta	F Ratio	Beta	F Ratio	Beta	F Ratio
Supervisor Support	-.14	(1.27)	-.05	(.40)	-.09	(.57)	-.05	(.43)	.10	(.97)	.06	(.96)
Worker Support	-.05	(.20)	-.02	(.05)	-.16	(2.16)	.10	(1.55)	.02	(.02)	.22	(12.16)***
Client Contact	.09	(.86)	-.09	(1.85)	.29	(9.43)*	.05	(.68)	.09	(1.14)	.06	(1.18)
Role Ambiguity	.18	(2.78)	.13	(2.79)	-.03	(.09)	.04	(.27)	-.00	(.00)	.03	(.28)
Role Conflict	-.19	(1.97)	-.04	(.18)	.14	(1.25)	-.09	(.06)	-.06	(.31)	-.08	(1.16)
Work Load	-.12	(.82)	.03	(.09)	.05	(.12)	.00	(.00)	-.22	(3.72)*	.07	(.82)
Intent to Quit	-.11	(.93)	.08	(1.05)	-.05	(.24)	-.15	(4.14)*	-.20	(4.17)*	-.10	(2.83)
Sex Discrimination	-.00	(.00)	.01	(.03)	-.18	(3.70)*	-.14	(3.95)*	-.28	(11.29)**	-.15	(7.95)**
Job Comfort	-.07	(.25)	.10	(1.11)	.25	(3.56)	-.06	(.32)	.05	(.16)	.21	(7.20)**
Financial Rewards	-.20	(3.27)	.09	(1.57)	-.00	(.00)	.07	(.89)	-.00	(.00)	-.07	(1.53)
Job Challenge	.17	(1.75)	.07	(.68)	.23	(3.59)	-.13	(2.53)	.20	(3.44)	.21	(11.00)***
	$R^2=.13$		$R^2=.07$		$R^2=.21$		$R^2=.07$		$R^2=.39$		$R^2=.42$	

* = < .05
** = < .01
*** = < .001

with clients, which was positively associated with increased depression.

The best predictors of irritation for both males and females was sex discrimination on the job, which was associated with increased irritation. The best predictors of irritation for females only were worker support, job comfort and work challenge, with a decreased likelihood of such factors associated with increased irritation. For males alone the best predictors of irritation were an increased work load and an increased intent to turn over.

An analysis of the zero-order correlation coefficients between these three psychological strain variables by gender, showed that for males no correlation coefficients exceeded .29, for females none exceeded .39, indicating a low to moderate relationship between these variables.

In order to determine the relative effects of the various job related predictors of the burnout variables, namely emotional exhaustion, depersonalization, and personal accomplishment, based upon the Maslach Burnout Inventory, we conducted a standardized multiple regression analysis for each of these subscales. The resulting beta weights, and F tests are presented in Table 4 for male and female workers.

The best predictor of emotional exhaustion for both males and females was intent to quit, in which an increased likelihood to quit was associated with increased emotional exhaustion. Some important differences between males and females emerged: for males, the most important predictor was increased amount of client contact which was associated with increased emotional exhaustion, but for females, the most important predictors of increased emotional exhaustion were decreased supervisor support, worker support, and job comfort.

The best predictor of depersonalization for both males and females was intent to quit, in which an increased likelihood to quit was associated with increased depersonalization. Some important gender differences emerged: for males a decreased likelihood of role ambiguity was associated with increased depersonalization, but for females the best predictors were a decreased amount of worker support and a less likelihood of challenge on the job, which were associated with increased depersonalization.

The best predictors of personal accomplishment for males and

Table 4

Job Facets as Predictors: Multiple Regression Analysis on Burnout Variables

Predictors	Emotional Exhaustion				Depersonalization				Personal Accomplishment			
	Males		Females		Males		Females		Males		Females	
	Beta	F Ratio	Beta	F Ratio	Beta	F Ratio	Beta	F Ratio	Beta	F Ratio	Beta	F Ratio
Supervisor Support	.13	(1.02)	-.15	(4.09)*	-.12	(1.15)	-.11	(2.51)	.13	(1.41)	.08	(1.21)
Worker Support	.11	(1.59)	.18	(6.23)**	.11	(1.06)	.24	(11.84)***	-.14	(1.84)	.01	(.04)
Client Contact	.18	(4.22)*	.06	(.98)	-.03	(.14)	.06	(1.08)	.19	(4.70)*	-.14	(6.03)**
Role Ambiguity	.08	(.76)	.08	(1.21)	.23	(5.17)*	-.11	(2.39)	-.08	(.61)	-.22	(9.47)**
Role Conflict	-.22	(3.53)	-.08	(.87)	.05	(.13)	-.15	(3.34)	.15	(1.49)	-.02	(.03)
Work Load	-.14	(1.49)	-.02	(.04)	.03	(.14)	.15	(3.56)	-.09	(.58)	-.12	(2.15)
Intent to Quit	-.29	(9.18)**	-.19	(7.94)**	-.24	(5.56)*	-.16	(5.75)**	-.00	(.00)	-.07	(1.27)
Sex Discrimination	-.02	(.07)	-.04	(.45)	-.00	(.00)	.06	(.80)	.12	(1.98)	.02	(.16)
Job Comfort	-.20	(2.86)	.17	(4.01)*	.13	(1.11)	.15	(3.18)	-.11	(.83)	-.18	(4.98)*
Financial Rewards	-.05	(.28)	-.02	(.09)	-.15	(2.11)	-.05	(.62)	.02	(.02)	.02	(.06)
Job Challenge	.12	(1.16)	.04	(.27)	.17	(2.00)	.20	(7.98)**	-.28	(5.73)**	-.32	(22.13)***
	$R^2=.33$		$R^2=.19$		$R^2=.24$		$R^2=.21$		$R^2=.28$		$R^2=.25$	

* = $<.05$
** = $<.01$
*** = $<.001$

females were increased client contact and job challenge. A greater likelihood of personal accomplishment was associated with increased client contact for men, and decreased client contact for women. An increase in job challenge was associated with increased personal accomplishment for both sexes. For females alone, the best predictors of personal accomplishment were a greater likelihood of job comfort and less role ambiguity. An analysis of the zero-order correlation coefficients between these three subscales showed that for males or females no correlation coefficients exceeded .43, indicating a low to moderate relationship between these dependent variables.

DISCUSSION

It is of interest that decreased emotional support from supervisors and co-workers was predictive of irritation, emotional exhaustion, and depersonalization for females, but not for males. These gender differences may reflect the findings by Pines, Aronson and Kafry (1981) that women may seek to cope with work stress by talking more about it with co-workers and may share more of their feelings than men, while men are more likely to have depersonalized feelings about the people they work with (Maslach, 1982). This gender difference may also be due to consequences of reported discomfort between the sexes in the area of collegial, social work relationships (Kadushin, 1976). Since more men (78%) than women (58%) in this sample are married, men may depend more upon spouses than upon supervisors and co-workers to fulfill their personal needs for affection and approval than women (Maslach, 1982). These considerations suggest that improvements in social support from co-workers and supervisors for both men and women, can be the target of interventions designed to increase opportunities for emotional support, friendships, and mutual approval in the work place to reduce the development of burnout and psychological strains.

Variables related to the stress of clinical work, such as the amount of time spent in such work, also present a gender differentiated picture. For women, increased contact with clients was associated with decreased personal accomplishment, while for men increased client contact was associated with increased depression, emotional exhaustion, and with an increased sense of personal accomplishment. These gender differences may reflect an ambivalent feeling toward increased client contact among men, which is supported by Kadushin's (1976) comment that most men may be expecting rapid advancement to administrative positions in social work agencies, and see prolonged involvement with clients as a barrier to the attainment of this goal. For women, increased client contact may reinforce the idea that administrative positions may not be open to them, or may reflect a dissatisfaction with increased levels of client work which makes intensive treatment of individuals less possible, due to a greater sense of involvement with people as stated in the literature (Maslach, 1982). Differential access to administrative positions by gender is also related to the issue of sex discrimination which will be discussed further.

Role ambiguity was also a significant predictor of burnout for men and women, with decreased role ambiguity associated with increased personal accomplishment for women, and with decreased role ambiguity associated with increased depersonalization for men. This latter gender difference underscores the previous comment concerning the uneasiness of men in the prescribed role of clinical worker. It is important, therefore, that male workers know what opportunities exist for advancement in social work settings, so that expectations and opportunities for such advancement are discussed with administrators and based upon the reality of the organizational structure.

Having an intent to quit a present job was an important stressor for both males and females. For males and females such an intent was associated with increased emotional exhaustion, and depersonalization, for females with increased depression, and for males with increased irritation. At some point, as Maslach (1982) has stated, clinical work becomes too much of a burden for professionals, and they may leave the field entirely or enter a different job within their field, typically one in administration. Therefore, it is of extreme importance that the causes of burnout and psychological strain be addressed early in the careers of clinical social workers, so that the idea of quitting the job, or the actual intention of quitting are minimized by attempts to relieve job stress. These attempts may include the development of ways of communicating with workers about job continuance and tenure. This type of discussion may permit work improvement to occur before the idea of quitting becomes a serious option for the individual.

Sex discrimination on the job was a significant predictor of increased depression and irritation for both men and women. Women reported a significantly higher mean score on this variable than men, but it obviously affects both sexes. These findings reflect the gender conflict which exists in a profession in which a majority of the workers are women, while administrative positions are held by a majority of men; and those men engaged in clinical work report dissatisfaction in their relationships with women co-workers (Kadushin, 1976; Fanshel, 1976). Sutton (1982) states that it is time that social workers admit to the fact that discriminating practices, especially toward women, exist within the profession, and that places of employment evaluate the fairness of their personnel policies and grievance procedures to promote better relationships among male and female workers.

Decreased job comfort is associated with increased irritation and depersonalization, and increased job comfort is associated with a greater sense of personal accomplishment for women only. Folkins, O'Reilly, Roberts, and Miller (1977) reported that an improved physical environment for work in a mental health center was associated with greater job satisfactions, but no gender differences were reported. Since in this study job comfort is an important issue for women, gender specific interventions need to be implemented to improve those aspects of travel to and from work, physical surroundings, and working hours which are a source of stress.

Financial rewards were not a significant predictor of burnout or psychological strains for either sex in this study, even though women reported significantly higher mean scores on this variable, indicating a greater dissatisfaction with pay, job security and fringe benefits. This finding is puzzling, since the literature supports the fact that women workers receive lower salaries than men, and is a source of serious concern among women workers (Fanshel, 1976; Sutton, 1982). This discrepancy may be due to a number of possibilities, namely that workers feel that they are coping adequately with this problem, or that other job stressors contribute more significantly to burnout and psychological strain, or that many workers are socialized to accept the pay levels in the profession. Further research is needed to examine this issue in the profession.

Increased job challenge was associated with increased personal accomplishment on the job for both men and women. A lesser likelihood of job challenge was associated with increased depersonalization and irritation for women. These findings support the contention made by Pines, Aronson and Kafry (1981) that one of the most common reasons for job dissatisfaction is the belief that work has no significance, and that the individual's potential for increased self-actualization and growth is not being stimulated. Therefore, it is important that the worker be given opportunities for the development of special abilities, the freedom to do tasks that are valued, and increased freedom to decide how a task should be accomplished, so that a sense of personal accomplishment can be increased and burnout and psychological strain reduced.

In conclusion, this study illustrates the increased specificity concerning the causes of burnout and psychological strain, which can result from the attention to gender differences in the effect of work stressors upon these factors. There are obvious gender differences in the reporting of the sources of work stress and in the manner of complaint about such stressors. Therefore, these gender differences require gender specific interventions targeted toward these differences. In this area of research investigation, as well, these differences need to be systematically investigated throughout the profession, rather than relying upon information based upon studies which ignore this gender issue. The reward will be a marked enrichment in the quality of the work environment, which will be perceived by both sexes.

REFERENCES

Barrett, M. & McKelvy, J. (1980). Stresses and strains of child welfare workers: Typologies for assessment. *Child Welfare, 59*, 277-285.

Berkeley Planning Associates (1977). *Evaluation of child abuse and neglect demonstration project, 1974-1977.* Berkeley, CA: Berkeley Planning Associates.

Caplan, R., Cobb, S., French, J., Van Harrison, R. & Pinneau, S. (1975). *Job demands and worker health.* Washington, DC: HEW.

Cohen, J. & Cohen, P. (1975). *Applied multiple regression/correlation analysis for the behavioral sciences*. Hillside, NJ: Lawrence Erlbaum Associates.
Fanshel, D. (1976). Status differentials: Men and women in social work. *Social Work, 21*, 448-454.
Folkins, C., O'Reilly, C., Roberts, K. & Miller, S. (1977). Physical environment and job satisfaction in a community mental health center. *Community Mental Health Journal, 31*, 24-30.
Freudenberger, H. (1977). Burn-out: Occupational hazard of the child care worker. *Child Care Quarterly, 56*, 90-99.
Harrison, W. (1980). Role strain and burnout in child protective service workers. *Social Service Review, 54*, 31-44.
Jayaratne, S. & Chess, W. (1983). Job satisfaction and burnout in social work. In B. Farber (ed.), *Stress and burnout in the human service professions*. New York: Pergamon Press, pp. 129-141.
Jayaratne, S., Tripodi, T. & Chess, W. (1983). Perceptions of emotional support, stress, and strain by male and female social workers. *Social Work Research and Abstracts, 19*, 19-27.
Justice, B., Gold, R. & Klein, J. (1981). Life events and burnout. *Journal of Psychology, 108*, 219-226.
Kadushin, A. (1976). Men in a woman's profession. *Social Work, 21*, 440-447.
Littner, N. (1974). The strains and stresses of the child welfare worker. *Child Welfare, 53*, 1-20.
Maslach, C. (1976). Burned-out. *Human Behavior, 15*, 16-22.
Maslach, C. (1982). *Burnout–The cost of caring*. Englewood Cliffs, NJ: Prentice Hall.
Maslach, C. & Jackson, S. (1981). The measurement of experienced burnout. *Journal of Occupational Behavior, 2*, 99-113.
Maslach, C. & Jackson, S. (1985). The role of sex and family variables in burnout. *Sex Roles, 12*, 837-851.
Maslach, C. & Pines, A. (1977). The burnout syndrome in the day care setting. *Child Care Quarterly, 6*, 100-133.
Morrow, L. (1981). The burnout of almost everyone. *Time Magazine*, September, p. 84.
Pines, A., Aronson, E. & Kafry, D. (1981). *Burnout: From tedium to personal growth*. New York: Free Press.
Pines, A. & Kafry, D. (1978). Occupational tedium in the social services. *Social Work, 23*, 499-507.
Quinn, R. & Sheppard, L. (1974). *The 1972-1973 quality of employment survey*. Ann Arbor, MI: Institute of Social Research.
Quinn, R. & Staines, G. (1978). *The 1975-1976 quality of employment survey*. Ann Arbor, MI: Institute of Social Research.
Rapoport, L. (1960). In defense of social work: An examination of stress in the profession. *Social Service Review, 34*, 62.
Rizzo, J. House, J. & Lirtzman, S. (1970). Role conflict and ambiguity in complex organizations. *Administrative Science Quarterly, 15*, 150-163.
Shinn, M., Rosario, M., March, H. & Chesnut, D. (1981). Coping with job stress and burnout in the human services. Manuscript. New York: New York University.
Sutton, J. A. (1982). Sex discrimination among social workers. *Social Work, 27*, 211-217.

The Association of Burnout and Social Work Practitioners' Impressions of Their Clients: Empirical Evidence

Kevin J. Corcoran

SUMMARY. This study examined the association between burnout and social work practitioners' impressions of their clients. The results provide empirical evidence that burnout adversely affects social work practice; emotional exhaustion and depersonalization were significantly correlated with negative impressions of clients.

Few topics in the social sciences have received enthusiasm parallel to burnout. Research, however, has lagged behind speculations and anecdotal accounts (Carroll & White, 1982). Even the definition of burnout is considered a vexing problem (Freudenberger, 1983; Corcoran, 1984).

This study examines one "self-evident" aspect of burnout; namely, the relationship between burnout and social work practitioners' impressions of their clients. As a secondary concern, the effect of client gender on social work practitioners' impression will be considered.

The primary concern of this research may seem moot and self-evident. In fact, from the time Freudenberger (1974) first introduced the term into the professional literature, numerous writers have asserted that burnout adversely affects the delivery of services. Maslach (1976) for example, has stated burnout "plays a major role in the poor delivery of health and welfare ser-

---

Dr. Corcoran is Assistant Professor, Graduate School of Social Work, University of Houston – University Park, Houston, TX 77004.

vices . . ." (p. 16). This effect is seen as reaching not only the individual worker and client, but the social service agency and non-work relationships, such as the worker's family (Jackson & Maslach, 1982). Pines and Aronson (1981, p. 15) see the effect in more general terms, relating burnout to negative attitudes towards others including clients. Maslach and Jackson (1981) further consider burnout in terms of "negative and cynical attitudes" (p. 2).

Maslach has more recently observed that most conceptualizations concern "a direct link between experienced burnout and a deterioration in the quality of services or care provided to clients" (1982, p. 40). This discussion was prefaced with "presumably," as there is insufficient empirical evidence, a contention also noted by Farber and Heifetz (1982).

This drawback is especially applicable to the relationship between burnout and clinical practice where research is generally scarce. In terms of the presumed association between burnout and an adverse effect on practice, little published research is available. One study suggests burned out workers consider themselves as having "difficulty" providing services (Streepy, 1981). This finding must be considered tentative as the researcher did not use a standardized measure of burnout and does not clarify what is meant by "difficulty" in providing services. No research was found in the author's search of the literature which directly examined how burnout is related to social work practice.

While burnout may adversely affect the practitioner's perception of the client, consideration must also be given to the client's gender. This variable has received considerable attention in terms of how gender affects psychotherapy (Lambert & Utic, 1982), clinical judgements and diagnosis (Sterns, Penner & Kimmel, 1980) and empathic communication (Eisenberg & Lennon, 1983) to mention a few areas pertinent to practice.

The effect of client gender has had mixed results in terms of its impact upon social work practitioners. Schwartz (1974), for example, found clinical workers to have a negative bias in evaluating their female clients. Fischer et al. (1976). however, found a pro-female bias among social workers, a finding not supported in Dailey's (1980) replication. Finally, Jayaratne and Irey (1981) surveyed the Academy of Certified Social Workers and found no substantive differences between the workers' perception of male and female clients. *Post hoc* analyses by Jayaratne and Irey did, however, reveal that female workers had more positive perceptions of female clients and more negative perceptions of male clients.

Since burnout is manifested as a negative attitude toward one's client, it is plausible that it is related to negative impressions of a client. In other words, the depersonalizing and cynical attitudes would be associated with clinician's perceiving the client more negatively. Consequently, it was hypothesized that burnout would be associated with social work practitioners' negative impressions of their clients. Secondly, it was hypothesized that practitioners would have more negative impressions of their male clients than female clients.

METHOD

Research Design and Procedures

Data collection occurred through a mailed survey. A test booklet was mailed to 300 randomly sampled female master level social workers from the Texas Chapter of the NASW. Approximately one month later a follow-up postcard was sent to all participants further requesting participation.

The test booklet included items assessing demographic information on the research participants and their "last or most recent client," measures of burnout and an assessment of their impression of a client; in terms of impression, participants were instructed to complete each item in reference to their "last or most recent client." This procedure followed that used by Jayaratne and Irey (1981). It specifically repeated the phrase three times with the intent to focus the research participant's attention on a single identified client.

Research Participants

Of the 300 female social workers sampled, 139 returned the questionnaires in usable form. This represents a response rate of

46.3%, which Babbie (1979) considers adequate for data analysis and is a generally high rate for survey of NASW members (Kirk & Fischer, 1976).

For the purpose of this study, only research participants whose employment was at least 50% in direct practice were defined as social work practitioners. Ninety-one participants met the criterion. An additional three respondents were dropped as their most recent client was either a group or a family. This resulted in sample of 88 practitioners. The sample averaged 39.2 years old ($sd = 10.79$), and the majority (61.5%) were either married or living with a permanent partner. The sample's human service related experience ranged from one to forty-three years, with a mean of 12.28 ($sd = 8.99$). The average number of client contact hours per week was 21.4 ($sd = 9.4$), which was primarily individual therapy ($\overline{X} = 11.39$, $sd = 8.68$) compared to group ($\overline{X} = 3.82$, $sd = 5.21$) or family therapy ($\overline{X} = 2.18$, $sd = 4.56$). These demographic variables reflect the state membership in terms of age, experience and mental status, which helps support the sample's representativeness in spite of the size.

Instrumentation

Burnout was defined by scores on two dimensions of the Maslach Burnout Inventory (MBI; Maslach & Jackson, 1981); namely, the 9-item Emotional Exhaustion subscale and 5-item Depersonalization subscale. While Maslach and Jackson (1981) report acceptable internal consistency and validity for each subscale, recent efforts to replicate the psychometrics have been discouraging for the subscale's orthogonality and the reliability of the depersonalization subscale (Caron, Corcoran & Simcoe, 1983; Krowinski, 1981). For the current sample, however, a reliability analysis using Cronbach's coefficient alpha was quite acceptable for the Depersonalization subscale ($\alpha = .84$) and the Emotional Exhaustion subscale ($\alpha = .89$).

Practitioners' impressions were operationalized by scores on the Impression scale (Jourard, 1971), an instrument used in research on self disclosure. The scale has 20 items with each presenting two polarized adjectives. Research participants were instructed to rate their impressions of their "last or most recent client." Currently, no published data are available on the Impression scale's reliability or validity.

RESULTS AND DISCUSSION

Measuring Practitioners' Impressions

As a consequence of the absence of psychometric data on the Impression scale, it was necessary to examine the instrument's structure and reliability. A principle component analysis of the 20 items resulted in five factors with eigenvalues exceeding 1.0. The first two factors accounted for slightly more than 50% of the variance. The remaining factors had only leniently acceptable eigenvalues (Cromrey, 1978), each accounting for less than 10% of the variance. These data, along with SCREE test, suggested that only the first two factors are meaningful summative subscales.

As displayed in Table 1, those items meeting the factor loading criterion of .40 (Nunnully, 1978) had simple structure using varimax rotation. The four items of the first factor seem to assess

Table 1

Factor Loadings for the Impression Scales

Item Content	Factor Loadings	
	Interpersonal	Intellectual
Warm-Cold	.863	-.067
Likeable-Unlikeable	.776	.259
Pleasant-Irritating	.739	.286
Considerate-Inconsiderate	.673	.095
Quit witted-Slowthinker	-.039	.859
Intelligent-Unintelligent	.097	.821
Attractive-Unattractive	.314	.641
Competent-Incompetent	.299	.623

an Interpersonal Impression of another, while the four items of the second factor appear to assess an Intellectual Impression. This factor analytic procedure may be seen as tentative support of the instrument's construct validity. The subscales' orthogonality is supported by their correlation ($r = .42$). The Interpersonal and Intellectual subscales each had acceptable reliability, with internal consistency coefficient of .84 and .83, respectively. The total Impression scale also had an acceptable *alpha* of .89.

In summary, the social work practitioners' impressions of their last or most recent client was ascertained through total scores on the Impression scale. In order to provide initial data on the specific nature of the practitioners' impressions, the Interpersonal Impression and Intellectual Impression subscales were included. For all measures higher scores indicate more negative impressions.

Burnout and Negative Impressions

Most studies have shown burnout to be associated with age and experience (Kafry, 1981). The data from this study support these findings for a sample of female social work practitioners. Age and experience were significantly correlated with both measures of burnout: age = $-.19$, $p < .05$ and $-.26$, $p < .01$; experience = $-.21$, $p < .05$ and $-.23$, $p < .05$. These findings suggest that as practitioners got older and gained more human service related experience they experienced less emotional exhaustion and depersonalization.

As a consequence of these findings, it was necessary to control for the participants' ages and experience in order to test the hypothesis of an association between burnout and practitioners' impressions. Pearson's correlations and partial correlations, with the variances due to age and experience removed, were used to test the hypothesis. These results are displayed in Table 2. The Pearson coefficients show a statistically significant association between both measures of burnout and practitioners' more negative impressions of their clients. These findings were consistent across all three impression measures, and remained statistically significant when social work practitioner's age and experience were partialled out.

Table 2

Pearson Correlations and Partial Correlations of
Social Work Practitioners' Burnout and Their Impressions of Clients

Burnout	Impressions Scales		
	Total	Interpersonal	Intellectual
Emotional Exhaustion	.34**	.26*	.30*
Controlling age	.31**	.26*	.26*
Controlling experience	.33**	.27*	.28*
Depersonalization	.31**	.24*	.33**
Controlling age	.28*	.25*	.28*
Controlling experience	.29*	.26*	.31**

*$p < .01$
**$p < .001$

These findings, thus, suggest two conclusions: one, that social work practitioners with higher levels of burnout have negative impressions of their clients; specifically, they had more negative impressions of clients interpersonally and intellectually. Secondly, the relationships between burnout and negative impressions are due neither to practitioner's age nor experience.

Difference Due to Client Gender

The data failed to support the second hypothesis of differences in social work practitioners' impressions as a result of client gender. The strongest difference was between male and female clients on the total Impression scale ($F [1, 77] = 2.08$) which was far from even approaching statistical significance.

The non-significant data fails to replicate previous findings (e.g., Fischer et al., 1976; Jayaratne & Irey, 1981) that female social workers have a negative bias against male and positive bias for female clients. One possible explanation for this may be the regional sample employed in this study compared to Jayaratne and Irey's national sample and Fischer et al.'s sample from Hawaii. The current sample was drawn from Texas, and it is possible that the average male who seeks treatment may somehow be different than the average male included in the other studies. Regardless of the speculations, the non-significant findings are encouraging as they suggest female social work practitioners do not have more negative impressions of their male clients than female clients.

CONCLUSIONS

In reviewing these findings, certain limitations must be considered. First of all, the sample was drawn from only one state and was small. Thus, the sample may have a regional bias and not be representative of the population of master level social workers. As far as the findings do represent the population, they are limited to female practitioners only.

Moreover, the findings may actually provide little insight into burnout. One reason is the correlational analyses which prohibit any assertion of causality. One interpretation of the finding is that burnout produced the more negative impressions of practitioners' clients. It is equally reasonable, however, that the impression scores were valid such that the clients warranted more negative impressions; if this is the case, such a client would likely be more difficult and stressful, thus resulting in higher levels of burnout among the practitioners. Future research will need to ferret out the directionality of this relationship.

In the meantime, the study provides empirical evidence to what Edelwich and Brodsky (1980) consider "the almost inevitable conclusions," that burnout affects clinical practice. Specifically, this study illustrated that social work practitioners had more negative impressions of their clients, seeing them more negatively interpersonally and intellectually. Moreover, these findings were not due to either the practitioners' ages or human service related experience. Finally, the findings further question the existence of a bias due to clients' genders.

REFERENCES

Babbie, Earl R. (1979). *The practice of social research*. 2nd ed. Belmont, CA: Wadsworth Publishing Company.
Caron, C., Corcoran, K. J. & Simcoe, F. (1983). Intrapersonal correlates of burnout: The role of locus of control in burnout and self-esteem. *The Clinical Supervisor, 1*(14), 53-62.
Carroll, J. F. X. & White, W. L. (1982). Theory building: Integrating individual and environmental factors within an ecological framework. In Whiton S. Paine (ed.), *Job stress and burnout: Research, theory and intervention perspectives*. Beverly Hills, CA: Sage, pp. 41-60.
Corcoran, K. J. (1986). Measuring burnout: A reliability and convergent validity study. *Journal of Social Behavior and Personality, 1*, 107-112.
Cromrey, A. L. (1978). Common methodological problems in factor analytic studies. *Journal of Consulting and Clinical Psychology, 46*(4), 648-659.
Dailey, D. M. (1980). Are social workers sexist: A replication. *Social Work, 25*, 45-50.
Edelwich, J. & Brodsky, A. (1980). *Burn-out: Stages of disillusionment in the helping professions*. New York: Human Sciences Press.
Eisenberg, N. & Lennon, R. (1983). Sex differences in empathy and related capacities. *Psychological Bulletin, 94*, 100-131.
Farber, B. A. & Heifetz, L. J. (1982). The process and dimensions of burn-out in psychotherapists. *Professional Psychology, 13*, 292-301.
Fischer, J., Dulaney, D. D., Fazior, R. T., Hudak, M. T. & Zivotofsky, E. (1976). Are social workers sexist? *Social Work, 21*, 428-433.
Freudenberger, H. J. (1983). Burnout: Contemporary issues, trends, and concerns. In B. A. Farber (ed.), *Stress and burnout in the human service professions*. New York: Pergamon Press, pp. 23-28.
Freudenberger, H. J. (1974). Staff burnout. *Journal of Social Issues, 1*, 159-164.
Jackson, S. E. & Maslach, C. (1982). After-effects of job-related stress: Families as victims. *Journal of Occupational Behavior, 3*, 63-77.
Jayaratne, S. & Irey, K. V. (1981). Gender differences in the perceptions of social workers. *Social Casework, 62*, 405-412.
Jourard, S. M. (1970). *Self disclosure: An experimental analysis of the transparent self*. New York: Wiley.
Kafry, D. (1981). The research, in A. M. Pines & E. Aronson, *Burnout: From tedium to personal growth*. New York: Free Press, pp. 202-222.
Kirk, S. A. & Fischer, J. (1976). Do social workers understand research? *Journal of Education for Social Work, 12*, 63-70.
Krowinski, W. J. (1981). A construct validation study of the Maslach Burn-out Inventory. Competency paper, University of Pittsburgh, School of Social Work.
Lambert, M. J. & Utic, J. (1982). Therapist characteristics and psychotherapy outcome. In M. J. Lambert (ed.), *The effects of psychotherapy*, volume 2. New York: Human Sciences Press.
Maslach, C. (1976). Burned-out. *Human Behavior, 5*, 16-22.
Maslach, C. (1982). *Burnout: The cost of caring*. Englewood Cliffs, NJ: Prentice-Hall.
Maslach, C. (1982). Understanding burnout: Definitional issues in analyzing a complex phenomenon. In W. S. Paine (ed.), *Job stress and burnout: Research, theory and intervention perspectives*. Beverly Hills, CA: Sage, pp. 29-40.

Maslach, C. & Jackson, S. E. (1981). The measurement of experienced burnout. *Journal of Occupational Behavior, 2*, 99-113.
Nunnally, J. (1978). *Psychometric theory*. New York: McGraw-Hill.
Pines, A. M. & Aronson, E., with Kafry, D. (1981). *Burnout: From tedium to personal growth*. New York: Free Press.
Schwartz, M. C. (1974). Importance of sex of worker and client. *Social Work, 19*, 177-185.
Sterns, B. C., Penner, L. A. & Kimmel, E. (1980). Sexism among psychotherapists: A case not yet proven. *Journal of Consulting and Clinical Psychology, 48*, 548-550.
Streepy, J. (1981). Direct-services providers and burnout. *Social Casework, 62*, 352-361.

Social Workers and Burnout: A Psychological Description

Mary Johnson
Gerald L. Stone

SUMMARY. This study explored different types of job stressors suggested by cognitive approaches to stress. The social work staff of several county social service agencies completed the Maslach Burnout Inventory, Work Environment Scale, the Jenkins Activity Survey and the Hassles Scale. The data were assessed for correlational trends using a modified hierarchical multiple regression model. Results of the study indicate that stress is related to the minor irritating events which characterize daily living. Additionally it was found that people who demonstrate Type A behavior patterns experience greater feelings of personal accomplishment.

Currently many writers are focusing on stress in occupational settings. Freudenberger (1974) and Maslach (1976) coined the term "burnout" to describe a particular kind of stress response experienced by those working in the helping professions such as social work. Burnout refers to a state of physical, emotional, and mental exhaustion resulting from involvement with people in emotionally demanding situations.

Most of the research on burnout (or job stress) has been limited by common sense notions or by the use of one particular theoretical framework. If one views stress primarily as a response to

---

Ms. Johnson is a doctoral candidate and an intern in professional psychology and Dr. Stone is Professor of Counseling Psychology, The University of Iowa. This study is based on a master's research project submitted by the senior author to the Counseling Psychology faculty at The University of Iowa. The second author served as the chief advisor to the senior author. Requests for reprints should be sent to Ms. Johnson, University Counseling Service, 101 Iowa Memorial Union, The University of Iowa, Iowa City, IA 52242.

© 1987 by The Haworth Press, Inc. All rights reserved.

external forces, then one is likely to be concerned about stimulus-defined sources of stress. For instance, past descriptive studies concerned with stress in a social work setting have focused on environmental variables (Daley, 1979; Harrison, 1980; Lowenberg, 1979; Mattingly, 1977; Pines & Kafry, 1978). If, on the other hand, one takes the interactional perspective suggested by recent literature (Lazarus & Folkman, 1984), the inclusion of cognitive processes in the determination of stress will become important.

In response to the recent emphasis on cognitive approaches to stress, the present descriptive study attended to psychological processes through the use of measures reflecting a more phenomenological or personalistic approach to stress. That is, each of the measures taps cognitive appraisal processes which help determine "daily hassles" (Hassles Scale), social climate of the work place (Work Environment Scale), personal response style (e.g., Type As, Jenkins Activity Scale), and job burnout (Maslach Burnout Inventory). Moreover, these measures can suggest different sources and types of stressors (little irritations, perceived environments, or personal characteristics) that may assist in efforts to understand and possibly reduce job stress within the helping professions.

METHOD

Participants

Participants consisted of 46 professional staff members (38 female and 8 male) of county social service agencies in the upper Midwest. The sample consisted of 31 social workers and 15 income maintenance (IM) workers. Social workers provided a full range of social services to their clientele, while the IM workers determined eligibility and dispersed federal, state and local aid to families with dependent children (AFDC) and relief funds. Due to sample size considerations, participants were combined across gender and worker type.

Procedure

Letters requesting volunteers were sent to eight county Social Service agencies serving similar client populations in rural communities. Out of a total population of 188 potential volunteers, 51 indicated an interest in participation. Volunteers were mailed four self-report measures which were packaged in random order. The completed measures were returned by mail. Of the original 51 packets mailed to volunteers, 37 were returned without follow-up within two weeks. Four more were returned after a postcard reminder and the last five were received after telephone contact. Five packets were not returned. Volunteers were advised in a cover letter that the questionnaires were intended to measure stress levels and that the measures were to be completed anonymously. Those who indicated an interest were offered written feedback about the results.

Measures

Maslach Burnout Inventory (MBI). The Maslach Burnout Inventory is composed of three subscales: (1) Emotional Exhaustion, (2) Depersonalization, and (3) Personal Accomplishment. Each subscale is measured by two dimensions, Frequency (range 1 to 6) and Intensity (range 1 to 7). The MBI was developed in a two-sage process on a combined sample of 1,025 persons in various human service occupations.

Internal consistency was estimated using Cronbach's alpha with data from the initial sample ($\alpha = .76$). Test-retest reliability data was obtained from a sample of graduate students (N = 53) for a 2-4 week interval ($r = .82$). Concurrent validity with behavioral ratings of MBI respondents by co-workers of 40 mental health workers had MBI scale scores which correlated moderately with co-workers' behavioral ratings of the respondents as burned-out (range from $r = .33$ to $r = .59$).

Hassles Scale. The Hassles Scale (Kanner, Coyne, Schaefer & Lazarus, 1981) is a 117-item questionnaire in which respondents are instructed to indicate the occurrence of any items which have "hassled" them in the past month. Participants rated each hassle on a 3-point scale as having been "somewhat," "moderately," or "extremely" severe. From this information, two scores are created: a frequency score, which is a count of the number of items checked, and an intensity score, which is the mean severity reported for all items checked. High scores reflect a greater number of hassles.

Items on the scale reflect the content areas of work (e.g., don't like work duties), family (e.g., not enough time for family), social activities (e.g., unexpected company), the environment (e.g., pollution), practical considerations (e.g., misplacing or losing things), finances (e.g., someone owes you money), and health (e.g., not getting enough rest).

Test-retest reliability over nine months is .79 for frequency and .48 for intensity. Construct validation coefficient with the Hopkins Symptom Checklist was found to be $r = .60$.

Work Environment Scale (WES). The Work Environment Scale assesses the social climate of work units. It focuses on three facets of the work setting: (1) interpersonal relationships among employees (Relationship Dimension); (2) the directions of personal growth emphasized in the work unit (Personal Growth Dimension); and (3) the basic organizational structure of the unit (System Maintenance and System Change Dimensions). High scores correspond with favorable impressions of the environment.

Moos and Insel (1974) report internal consistency coefficients ranging from .70 to .91. Also several recent studies (e.g., Rosenthal, Teague, Retish, West & Vessell, 1983) found worker perceptions (WES) to be highly correlated with job stress.

Jenkins Activity Survey (JAS). Type A behavior patterns were determined by responses to the Jenkins Activity Survey. The JAS is a 21-item, self-administered, hand-scored questionnaire. A score of nine or above (range 0-21) indicates Type A personality. The JAS was validated on a sample of 419 coronary heart disease victims. It identified 72% of the group that had been diagnosed Type A following an interview (Jenkins, Zyzanski & Rosenman, 1971). The 21 items of the JAS measure Type A behavior and three other factors associated with the pattern: (1) Hard-Driving Competitiveness, (2) Speed and Impatience, and (3) Job Involvement. Test-retest reliability over six months was .91.

RESULTS

Preliminary Analyses

The first step in the data analyses was to obtain the means and standard deviations of the variables (see Table 1). Pearson product-moment correlations were then computed (see Table 2). These correlations were based on the sample of 46 respondents.

Table 1

Sample Description

Variable	M	SD	Range
Age	37	7.75	26-59 years
Years in Current Position	6.3	7.90	.16-18 years
Years in This Type of Work	11.0	8.0	.41-24 years
Hassles	32.9	19.9	0-117
Jenkins Activity Survey	9.0	3.5	0-21
Work Environment Scale			
Relationship	13.7	5.9	0-27
Growth	10.0	3.2	0-18
System	23.6	5.4	0-45
Burnout			
Emotional Exhaustion			
Frequency	26.8	11.9	0-54
Intensity	34.8	11.9	0-63
Depersonalization			
Frequency	9.3	6.0	0-33
Intensity	12.4	6.9	0-35
Personal Accomplishment			
Frequency	35.3	7.1	0-48
Intensity	38.6	7.1	0-56

Table 2

Pearson Correlation Coefficients

	Burnout	Personal Accomplishment	Age	Exp	Ed	JAS	Hassles	REL	WES Growth	Systems
Burnout										
Personal Accomplishment	.079									
Age	.054	-.103								
Exp	-.392*	-.140	.229							
Ed	-.045	.138	-.125	.004						
JAS	.129	.549**	-.163	.161	.010					
Hassles	.583**	.023	-.129	-.085	.226*	.148				
REL	-.117	.364	-.092	.037	-.037	.311	-.051			
Growth	.133	.375	-.045	-.238*	-.206	.333	.023	.614**		
System	.072	.194	.173	-.218	-.227	.180	-.145	.313*	.525**	

*p ≤ .05   Exp = Experience   JAS = Jenkins Activity Survey   Growth = Personal growth dimension
**p ≤ .001 Ed = Education   WES = Work Environment Scale   System = System maintenance
                              REL = Relationship dimension   system change dimension

The descriptive analysis yielded an average profile of a 37-year-old, married female with a bachelor's degree and 11 years of experience in social work (see Table 1). Overall, the respondents in this study were experiencing moderate levels of job stress as measured by the MBI. The scores all fell within the "moderate" range relative to a normative sample of 2,118 persons reported by the authors of the MBI. The norm sample included members of a variety of helping professions, including social workers.

Data reduction analysis was undertaken due to the small sample size. These analyses revealed a substantial interrelationship between the Emotional Exhaustion and Depersonalization subscales (including both the frequency and intensity dimensions) on the MBI (see Table 3). As a result, a linear combination of these scales was completed. This constituted the criterion variable, burnout. A second criterion variable, personal accomplishment, was then formed from a similar linear combination of the frequency and intensity dimension of the third MBI subscale, Personal Accomplishment. It was conceptualized as a positive index, providing additional information to the traditional burnout index, although caution is recommended in using this index because of the limited sample size.

Four independent variables were selected. The first independent variable cluster consisted of the demographic variables of age, level of education and years of experience. These variables have been shown to be empirically related to job stress in previous research (Maslach & Jackson, 1981). The three primary independent variables consisted of the single score indexes from the JAS and the Hassles (frequency) Scale, and a derived score from the WES. The frequency dimension of the Hassles Scale was selected because previous research identifies it as the most cogent of the potential indexes (Kanner, Coyne, Schaefer & Lazarus, 1981). The WES consists of ten subscales which are organized around three empirically derived dimensions: Relationship, Personal Growth and System Maintenance, and System Change (Moos & Insel, 1974). A moderate interrelationship was found in this study, among the scales within each dimensionon the WES. This is consistent with previous research and it lends further support to the existence of these dimensions. Summative scores for

Table 3

Correlation Coefficients MBI Subscales

Scale	EEF	EEI	DPF	DPI	PAF	PAI
Emotional Exhaustion						
Frequency (EEF)						
Intensity (EEI)	.806**					
Depersonalization						
Frequency (DPF)	.675**	.471**				
Intensity (DPI)	.553**	.611**	.653**			
Personal Accomplishment						
Frequency (PAF)	.10	-.021	.060	.160		
Intensity (PAI)	-.09	.038	-.186	-.102	.620**	

*p ≤.05

**p ≤.001

the three dimensions were constructed from the subscales within each dimension in order to reduce the overall number of variables which would be entered in subsequent analyses.

In summary, the data reduction analyses yielded two dependent variables (burnout, personal accomplishment), three primary independent variables (WES, JAS, Hassles), and one control independent variable cluster representing age, level of education, and years of experience.

In the next step a modified hierarchical multiple regression (Cohen & Cohen, 1975) was used to investigate the relationship between the criterion variables and the independent variables. A separate regression analysis was run on each dependent variable because of their statistical and conceptual independence (Maslach & Jackson, 1981). In a modified hierarchical procedure the unique contribution of each independent variable to the total variance of the dependent variable can be determined when each independent variable is systematically added last to the regression model. This process does not solve the problem of multicolinearity, although the clustering of variables may reduce its effect. Multicolinearity is an important issue here as the WES was found to have a relationship with the JAS, suggesting some degree of overlap on these independent variables. Descriptive variables were entered first in each regression model so that the effects of more interesting variables could be examined in terms of what they add by way of explanation/prediction. After this initial entry in each of the subsequent analyses, each independent variable was assessed as it was entered last in a stepwise progression.

Outcome Analyses

The results of the regression analyses are listed in Table 4 where the amount of unique variance accounted for by each variable is listed. Overall, results indicate that 50 percent of the variance in burnout could be explained by the control and primary independent variables ($F = 3.71, p < .01$). The Hassles Scale alone accounts for a significant amount of the total variance in burnout (25%; $F = 16.81, p < .001$). The other independent variables do not make significant contributions (JAS = 2%, WES = 3%, Control = 13%).

In the second analysis, the independent and control variables account for 38% of the variance in personal accomplishment ($F = 2.32, p < .05$). A significant amount of the total variance in feelings of personal accomplishment is accounted for by the JAS (17%, $F = 9.05, p < .01$). Contributions of the other variables were not significant (WES = 6%, Hassles = 0%, Control = 5%) when entered last.

In summary, burnout is related to the chronic hassles of daily living, however minor, from many sources over a long period of time. Additionally, feelings of personal accomplishment appear to be associated with the Type A personality.

DISCUSSION

Major Findings

The results reveal a significant relationship (although the clinical significance of the magnitude is debatable) between burnout

Table 4

Regression Analysis Summary

Cluster/Variable	Job Stress $R^2\Delta$	Job Stress F	Personal Accomplishment $R^2\Delta$	Personal Accomplishment F
Control[1]	.133	1.46	.054	.60
Age	.002	1.88	.011	.49
Months in Current Position	.004	3.24	.022	.00
Months in Type of Work	.124	3.81	.022	2.21
Education	.001	0.11	.004	.45
Hassles	.253	16.81**	.002	0.09
Work Environment Scale[1]	.028	2.34	.061	2.32
Relationship	.019	1.80	.059	1.88
Personal Growth	.008	0.52	.001	0.08
System Maintenance	.001	0.03	.001	0.61
System Change				
Jenkins Activity Survey	.019	1.27	.168	9.05*

Note[1]. The variables in this cluster were entered using a forward selection procedure.

Note[2]. Table entries reflect the amount of unique variance accounted for.

*$p \leq .01$

**$p \leq .001$

and the relatively minor unpleasant events which accumulate and characterize daily living. These results are consistent with other research findings which link daily hassles to depression (Lewinsohn & Talkington, 1979), and overall health status (DeLongis, Coyne, Dakof, Folkman & Lazarus, 1982). The direction of causes in a correlational relationship is always problematic.

These findings therefore could support both the contention that occupational stress can affect one's sensitivity to minor, daily hassles, as well as the contention that the effect of repeated minor daily annoyances are additive over time and impact larger psychological systems (e.g., interpersonal relationships, self-esteem, and others). The establishment of a direct causal linkage between burnout and hassles requires further empirical examination.

Another suggestive finding is the significant relationship between Type A behavior patterns and feelings of personal accomplishment. This finding is contrary to other research which highlights the negative psychological effects experienced by Type A personalities. Type A personalities are described as being competitive, impatient, easily provoked, having excessive drive and hostility. Here the emphasis is on the positive aspects of Type A personality.

Although correlational data is insufficient for strong inferences about the nature of the relationship between Type A characteristics and personal accomplishments, the finding does seem to fit recent research on self-efficacy (Bandura, Adams & Beyer, 1977) and the literature on achievement-oriented Type A personalities. Both literatures suggest that individuals with such characteristics will seek out opportunities and attempt tasks related to personal accomplishment and, therefore, are likely to identify and experience personal accomplishment when it occurs.

A final outcome of this exploratory study is the suggested range of stressors that may need to be considered in identifying the nature of job stress. These include environmental, intrapersonal, and interactional stressors.

Limitations

The interpretability of this study is limited by features of the sample (size, representativeness, variability), the measures (self-report, psychometric soundness), and the design (correlational). Additionally other unstudied variables may be operating. Intrapersonal variables (coping skills, beliefs) may help determine the subjective appraisal of the significance of an event. Individual differences in the availability of support or personal resources might also impact the relation between burnout and daily hassles. Finally, features of the harassing events may be implicated. Is it the number, duration, frequency, or expectedness of the hassle that triggers stress? Is it the actual nature of the hassle (i.e., reporting requirements, range of client difficulties that must be dealt with, and others) that interacts with psychological vulnerabilities? Or is the possible absence of offsetting positive experiences involved? The answers to these questions have practical as well as theoretical significance.

Implications

Burnout research has as its ultimate objective the amelioration of the negative effects of stress. Although we do not clearly understand the relationship between burnout and daily hassles, the findings of this study suggest some intervention guidelines. These guidelines can be used by individuals, by work groups, and/or in administrative planning.

- First Step: The most logical initial step is to identify significant daily hassles. This can be done either through a personal inventory or in discussion with others who share the same environment.
- Second Step: This step may include simply acknowledging common annoyances and accepting their inevitability or it may include a systematic reduction of the harassment effect. A system for reducing harassment might include establishing a means for recognizing personal accomplishment or structuring for offsetting positive experiences. Specific solutions can be generated individually or within the work environment by providing coping skill education.
- Third Step: The final step is to periodically reassess hassles and stress levels given the changing nature of people and environments.

The object of these guidelines is to alter the subliminal nature of hassles and reduce the cumulative negative effects. There is certainly no such thing as a stress or hassle-free environment.

However, it may be possible to induce a greater sense of personal control and efficacy when job stress/hassles are recognized.

In summary, the stress experienced by the social workers in this study appears to be related to the minor irritating events which accumulate and characterize daily living. There does not appear to be a substantial relationship between stress and features of the work environment or specific aspects of the individual's personality. When these findings are compared with other research findings we may discover that burnout is not a unitary concept but rather that it assumes different dimensions in different occupations. Whatever the outcome, it is clear that burnout is a complex and varied phenomenon and our understanding of it is only beginning.

REFERENCES

Bandura, A., Adams, N. E. & Beyer, J. (1977). Cognitive processes mediating behavioral change. *Journal of Personality and Social Psychology, 35*, 125-139.

Cohen, J. & Cohen, P. (1975). *Applied multiple regression/correlational analysis for the behavioral sciences*. Hillsdale, NJ: Lawrence Erlbaum.

Daley, M. R. (1979). Burnout: Smoldering problem in protective services. *Social Work, 24*, 375-379.

DeLongis, A., Coyne, J., Dakof, G., Folkman, S. & Lazarus, R. (1982). Relationship of daily hassles, uplifts, and major life events to health status. *Health Psychology, 1*, 119-136.

Freudenberger, J. H. (1974). Staff burn-out. *Journal of Social Issues, 30*, 159-165.

Harrison, D. (1980). Role strain and burnout in child-protection service workers. *Social Service Review, 54*, 31-44.

Jenkins, C. D., Zyzanski, S. J. & Rosenman, R. H. (1971). Progress toward validation of a computer scored test for the Type A coronary-prone behavior pattern. *Psychosomatic Medicine, 33*, 193-202.

Kanner, A., Coyne, J., Schaefer, C. & Lazarus, R. (1981). Comparison of two modes of stress measurement: Daily hassles and uplifts versus major life events. *Journal of Behavioral Medicine, 4*, 1-23.

Lazarus, R. S. & Folkman, S. (1984). *Stress, appraisal, and coping*. New York: Springer.

Lewinsohn, P. M. & Talkington, J. (1979). Studies of the measurement of unpleasant events and relations with depression. *Applied Psychological Measurement, 3*, 101.

Lowenberg, F. M. (1979). Causes of turnover among social workers. *Journal of Sociology and Social Welfare, 6*, 622-641.

Maslach, C. (1976). Burned-out. *Human Behavior, 5*, 16-22.

Maslach, C. & Jackson, S. (1981). The measurement of experienced burnout. *Journal of Occupational Behavior, 2*, 1-15.

Mattingly, M. (1977). Sources of stress and burn-out in professional child care work. *Child Care Quarterly, 6*, 107-137.

Moos, R. & Insel, P. M. (1974). *Combined preliminary manual, family, work and group environment scales*. CA: Consulting Psychologists Press.

Pines, A. & Kafry, D. (1978). Occupational tedium in the social services. *Social Work, 23*, 499-507.

Rosenthal, D., Teague, M., Retish, P., West, J. & Vessell, R. (1983). The relationship between work environment attributes and burnout. *Journal of Leisure Research, 15*(2), 125-135.

Burnout Among Social Workers Working with Physically Disabled Persons and Bereaved Families

Ariela Stav
Victor Florian
Esther Zernitsky Shurka

SUMMARY. The present study investigated and compared the professional burnout level of rehabilitation social workers working in different rehabilitation agencies. The burnout level measured in the three groups of rehabilitation social workers was also compared to the burnout level experienced by a group of social workers working in social welfare agencies. One hundred and twelve subjects filled out the Maslach Burnout Inventory (MBI). The MBI consists of four factors: Emotional exhaustion, Depersonalization, reduced Personal Accomplishment and Personal Involvement, each of which is independently scored. The instrument also assesses both the frequency and intensity of the feelings represented by each of the factors. The results demonstrated that there were differences in manifestations and sources of burnout among the four groups. These differences are discussed in relation to job setting variables.

In recent years the effects of the burnout phenomenon on performance of the helping professions in various health, welfare and rehabilitation services has been widely discussed in the professional literature (Cherniss, 1980a; Edelwich & Brodsky, 1980; Emener, 1979; Emener, Luck & Gohs, 1982; Freudenberger, 1980; Maslach & Jackson, 1981).

Ms. Stav is Supervisor of Social Services, Haifa Rehabilitation Department, Ministry of Defence, Haifa, Israel, Dr. Florian is Senior Lecturer and Dr. Shurka is Lecturer, School of Social Work, University of Haifa, Mount Carmel, Haifa, Israel. Requests for reprints should be addressed to Ms. Stav.

© 1987 by The Haworth Press, Inc. All rights reserved.

Burnout is described as a multifaceted and cumulative process that involves many variables related to the work setting, the worker's personality, and the characteristics of clients and their problems (Cherniss, 1980; Daley, 1979; Emener, 1979; Freudenberger, 1980; Maslach & Jackson, 1982). The interaction among the above variables may lead to tension and stress that can result in the burnout phenomenon. Emener and Luck (1980) give a vivid illustration of the burned-out person as

> ... one who has lost his or her concern and enthusiasm for the organization, co-workers, goals and purposes of the job and the customers or consumers of the goods and services of the organization. Burnout persons are frequent complainers who view all ideas and suggestions in a sour, or a pessimistic way. They are resentful, disenchanted, fatigued, bored, discouraged, confused, edgy, quick to anger and frustrated over items of mild importance or relevance (p. 139).

One of the main factors contributing to burnout is the client's specific characteristics and problems. Rehabilitation clients constitute a unique group due to the chronic nature of their condition. Few studies have dealt with clients in chronic conditions and their effects on variables leading to professional burnout. Existing research has found that working with mentally retarded persons (Sarata, 1972), psychiatric clients (Cherniss & Egnatios, 1978), alcohol abusers (Valle, 1979), cystic-fibrosis patients (Lewiston, Conley & Blessing-Moore, 1981) and deaf children (Meadow, 1981) involves frustrations about how time is spent, dissatisfaction with treatment outcomes and feelings of guilt about professional failure. These negative expressions are all strongly conducive to burnout.

People with chronic illnesses and physical disabilities constitute a significant proportion of rehabilitation clients. Relatively little empirical data have been reported about burnout among professionals working with these rehabilitation groups (Florian & Shurka, 1986; Rigar, Harrington-Godley & Hafer, 1984). Maslach (1978) and Maslach and Jackson (1982) observed that in many situations it is the "chronics" that cause the most emotional stress for the staff. Professionals often feel less equipped to repeatedly handle the more mundane problems of clients who won't go away or never seem to show signs of improvement. Moreover, Faffer (1981) stated that in treating persons with serious disabilities, which affected their capacities in other life areas, professionals expressed difficulty in dealing with such feelings as the client's loss of desire to live and suicidal intentions.

Research on loss has demonstrated similarity between the psychological reactions and emotions evoked by physical disability and bereavement (Alexy, 1980; Falek & Britton, 1974; Hughes, 1980; Orfirer, 1970; Parkes, 1975; Wright, 1983). In both states clients go through similar psychological experiences in the various stages related to the process of reaction to loss. Thus, it may be assumed that professionals working in rehabilitation with bereaved families will undergo the same kinds of pressure as those working with physically disabled persons: this is the same pressure that is described as being related to professional burnout (Maslach & Jackson, 1982).

Most of the rehabilitation agencies in Israel are governmental and centralized. The two major agencies are the Ministry of Defense (MOD) and the National Insurance Institute (NII). The MOD offers separate rehabilitation services to two different groups of clients: disabled veterans and bereaved families of fallen soldiers. The NII (an institution parallel to Social Security in the US) offers rehabilitation services to persons with disabilities from the civilian sector, and also to those families who have experienced the loss of a family member due to work accidents. One of the major differences between the two agencies is that in the MOD a clear differentiation is made between the rehabilitation services offered to veterans with physical disabilities and those given to bereaved families. In the NII, the same social worker usually deals with both kinds of rehabilitation. Besides these two major agencies, there are governmental social welfare agencies that are divided according to regional areas to deliver social services to a diverse population. Social workers working within these agencies apply a predominately generic approach in service delivery. In contrast to the previously mentioned major agencies, social welfare agencies deal with a wide range of social, economical, familial and emotional problems. In this context, it is important to emphasize that all these rehabilitation agencies are usually part of a rigid bureaucratic framework—something which acts as an additional element of pressure that increases the individual worker's feeling of stress (Emener, 1979).

The purpose of the present study was to examine the burnout level among rehabilitation social workers as compared to welfare agency social workers. Two main hypotheses were formulated:

1. The burnout level of social workers in rehabilitation agencies will be higher than the burnout level of social workers in welfare agencies.
2. There will be differences in the burnout level between rehabilitation social workers in the framework of the NII and rehabilitation social workers in the MOD.

METHOD

Subjects

In Israel, in contrast to the U.S., rehabilitation counseling does not exist as a profession. Most of the rehabilitation work is performed by social workers with at least a BA degree in social work. Thus the subjects in the present study consisted of 112 social workers divided into four groups:

A. Twenty-nine MOD social workers who represented the entire population working with physically disabled veterans.
B. Twenty-three MOD social workers who constituted the entire population working with bereaved families.
C. Thirty randomly chosen NII social workers working with physically disabled persons and bereaved families from the civilian sector.
D. A control group consisting of 30 randomly chosen social workers in social welfare agencies.

In order to control the variables of gender and work experience, the sample was restricted to females who had worked for at least one year in the same agency. The results of a chi-square test showed no significant differences among the four groups in the demographic characteristics of age, ethnic origin, educational background and work experience.

Instruments

The main instrument of the present study was the Maslach Burnout Inventory (MBI—Maslach & Jackson, 1981). The MBI consists of 22 items designed to measure hypothetical aspects of the burnout syndrome (Maslach & Jackson, 1981). The items are written in the form of statements about personal feelings or attitudes.

Each statement is rated on two dimensions—frequency and intensity. The frequency scale ranges from 0 ("never") to 6 ("every day"). The intensity scale ranges from 0 ("never") to 7 ("major, very strong"). Factor analysis of the 22 items based on a total sample of $N = 1025$ using principal factoring with interaction plus an orthogonal rotation, yielded a three factor solution. The factors that emerged were similar for both the frequency and the intensity ratings:

1. The Emotional Exhaustion subscale describes the feelings of being emotionally overextended and exhausted by one's work (9 items).
2. The Depersonalization subscale describes a lack of feeling and impersonal response towards recipients of one's care or service (5 items).

For both these subscales a higher mean scores indicates a higher level of burnout.

3. The Personal Accomplishment subscale assesses feelings of competence and successful achievement in one's work with people (8 items). In contrast to the above two subscales, lower mean scores on this subscale correspond to higher levels of burnout.

The authors reported that internal consistency was estimated by Cronbach's alpha coefficient. The internal reliability coefficients for the subscales range from .71 to .76 ($p < .001$) for frequency and from .76 to .87 ($p < .001$) for intensity. The test-retest reliability coefficients ranged from .60 to .82 for frequency and from .53 to .69 for intensity and were also significant beyond the .001 level. The authors reported a high level of concurrent validity, construct validity and discriminant validity (see data Maslach & Jackson, 1981).

For the purpose of this study, the MBI was specially translated into Hebrew by three social science professionals. The final version was based on total agreement between the translators. A pretest of the Hebrew scale on a sample of 24 social workers yielded a Cronbach alpha reliability coefficient of .68. The means and standard deviations obtained for each subscale were similar to those reported by Maslach and Jackson (1981). Based on Cherniss's (1980b) suggested list of stress provoking job-setting variables, subjects filled a brief questionnaire describing characteristics of their work setting, such as caseload, time allocation, supervision and bureaucratic intervention.

In addition to the MBI, subjects filled out a short demographic questionnaire based on the format of the Maslach and Jackson study.

Procedure

After the supervisors in each agency were initially contacted, special meetings were organized of staff members for the purpose of data collection. At these meetings a general explanation about the questionnaires was given and subjects were asked to fill out the research instrument, in small groups (between 8-10). Completion of the questionnaires took between 40-50 minutes. All the subjects who were contacted agreed to participate in the study.

RESULTS

The means and standard deviations for each MBI subscale in the four research groups are presented in Table 1. In order to test possible dependence among the subscales an overall MANOVA analysis, using Wilks criterion, was performed. This analysis revealed a significant difference among the

TABLE 1

Means and Standard Deviations of the Four Research Groups on the M.B.I*

Research groups Burnout Factors		M O D Rehab. Social Workers with Bereaved Families		M O D Rehab Social Workers with Physi- cally Dis- abled Veterans		N I I Rehab. Social workers with Bereaved Families and Physically Disabled Persons		Social Workers in Social Welfare Agencies	
		N=23		N=29		N=30		N=30	
		X	S.D.	X	S.D.	X	S.D.	X	S.D.
Emotional	Frequency	2.35	0.74	2.55	0.92	2.33	0.83	2.04	0.85
Exhaustion	Intensity	3.73	1.05	3.65	1.22	3.22	0.78	3.17	1.30
Depersonalization	Frequency	1.09	0.75	1.35	0.84	1.27	0.91	0.99	0.56
	Intensity	2.16	1.64	2.04	1.37	1.83	0.95	1.70	1.20
Personal Accomplishment	Frequency	3.38	0.74	4.12	0.57	3.96	0.70	3.63	0.99
	Intensity	4.79	0.76	5.00	0.51	4.49	0.60	4.65	0.77
Personal Involvement	Frequency	2.37	0.90	2.20	0.89	2.30	0.96	1.58	0.84
	Intensity	3.91	1.20	3.44	1.24	3.24	1.18	2.63	1.15

* The score range is 1-6 in the Frequency dimension and 1-7 in the Intensity dimension.
A high score means a high burnout level in the Emotional Exhaustion, Depersonalization and Personal Involvement Factors, while the opposite is the case for the Personal Accomplishment Factor.

research groups on specific factors (F = 1.98; df = 24, 293; p < .005). In order to identify which factors contributed to the differences among the groups, a one-way ANOVA was performed for each factor separately. This analysis revealed:

- significant differences among the groups on the intensity dimension of the personal accomplishment factor (F = 3; df = 3, 108; p < .03). A contrast analysis using Duncan's Multiple Range Test revealed that the MOD rehabilitation social workers, working with physically disabled veterans, showed the lowest burnout level, while NII rehabilitation social workers, working with both civilian physically disabled persons and bereaved families, showed the highest level of burnout.
- significant differences among the groups on the frequency dimension of the personal involvement factor (F = 4.5; df = 3, 108; p < .005). A contrast analysis using Duncan's Multiple Range Test revealed that the social workers in social welfare agencies showed the lowest burnout level compared to the other three research groups.
- significant differences among the groups on the intensity dimension of the personal involvement factor (F = 5.26; df = 3, 108; p < 0.02). A contrast analysis using Duncan's Multiple Range Test revealed that the social workers in social welfare agencies showed the lowest burnout level, both groups of MOD rehabilitation social workers showed the highest level of burnout while NII social workers did not significantly differ from these two subsets.

The next stage of the analysis of the data examined possible differences among the four groups according to job setting variables. Table 2 presents the means and standard deviations of the five job setting variables.

Based on a one-way ANOVA analysis the five job setting variables we found to be statistically significant are:

- *Caseload:* (F = 8.9; df = 3, 94; p < 0.0001). A Duncan Multiple Range Test revealed that MOD rehabilitation so-

TABLE 2
Means and Standard Deviations of the Four Research Groups on the Work Setting Variables

Research groups / Work Setting Variables	M O D Rehab. Social Workers with Bereaved Families		M O D Rehab. Social Workers with Physically Disabled Veterans		N I I Rehab. Social workers with Bereaved Families and Physically Disabled Persons		Social Workers in Social Welfare Agencies	
	N=23		N=29		N=30		N=30	
	X	S.D.	X	S.D.	X	S.D.	X	S.D.
Caseload	20.80	10.40	29	8.80	19.00	10.50	17.10	8.00
Percentage of time for Staff Consultation	20.20	10.02	19.31	6.30	15.70	7.53	23.10	8.50
Percentage of Time for Job Supervision	11.70	5.80	11.37	5.40	10.70	8.81	5.20	4.90
Satisfaction with Supervision 1-3 (1=High; 3=Low)	1.68	0 70	1.37	0 56	2.14	0.7	2.05	0.77
Bureaucratic Intervention 1-3 (1=High;3=Low)	2.43	0.50	1.86	0 74	2.23	0.60	2.00	0.70

cial workers, working with physically disabled veterans had the heaviest caseload compared to the other three groups.

— *Staff Consultation:* (F = 3.6; df = 3, 94; p < 0.01). A Duncan Multiple Range Test revealed that social workers in social welfare agencies spent more time in staff consultations compared to all social workers while both groups of MOD social workers did not differ significantly from either of these two subsets.

— *Job Supervision:* (F = 3.9: df = 3, 94; p < 0.01). A Duncan Multiple Range Test revealed that both groups of MOD social workers spent more time in receiving job supervision compared to welfare agency social workers, while the NII

social workers did not differ significantly from either of these two subsets.
- *Satisfaction with Supervision:* (F = 7.08; df = 3, 94; p < 0.0003). A Duncan Multiple Range Test revealed that MOD social workers working with disabled veterans showed the highest level of satisfaction compared to NII and social agency social workers, who showed the lowest level of satisfaction while the MOD social workers, working with bereaved families fell between these subsets.
- *Bureaucratic Intervention:* (F = 3; df = 3, 94; p < 0.03). A Duncan Multiple Range Test revealed the MOD social workers working with disabled veterans reported the highest level of bureaucratic intervention compared to MOD social workers, working with bereaved families, while neither of the other two research groups differed significantly from the two subsets.

The last step in the analyses of the data examined the possible relationship between job setting variables and the different burnout factors. A Multiple Regression analysis failed to show any significant relationship between these two sets of variables. In addition a correlation matrix was performed and from the 40 possible correlations (5 × 4 × 2), only four correlations reached a level of statistical significance. However, all these significant correlations were low (.19 to .28), possibly reaching significant levels as a result of the size of the sample (n = 112).

DISCUSSION

This research was initiated in light of the increasing interest in the burnout phenomenon that has become common among professionals working directly with clients. This phenomenon may result in a significant change in social workers' perception of their clients and their own capacity for providing adequate professional help (Maslach & Jackson, 1981). The purpose of the present study was to examine different dimensions of burnout experience by Israeli social workers in different job settings which deal with clients who experienced a condition of loss.

In general, the results revealed burnout scores that were relatively lower in comparison to those reported in research carried out in the United States (Maslach & Jackson, 1981). Similar findings have been reported in several other studies (Eldar, 1981; Etzion, Kafry & Pines, 1982; Kafry & Pines, 1980; Pines, Aronson & Kafry, 1981). The authors of these studies explained their findings by citing sociocultural factors and the unique character and structure of Israeli society. They stated that the greater emphasis on social unity and informality in interpersonal relations in Israel provided a sound basis for the creation of a social support system. In the U.S., on the other hand, the emphasis on competitiveness, excellence, and personal achievement may have contributed to feelings of guilt and anxiety that augment the burnout process.

In view of the relatively low scores of all four of the research groups, it is difficult to pinpoint broad differences among them. However, the results show that the rehabilitation social workers indicated higher burnout scores on the personal involvement factor in comparison with the social welfare agency workers (see Table 1). It appears that personal involvement is inevitable for these workers who spend their time dealing with problems of physical disability or death, situations that have a universal relevance and might threaten each worker personally. Emener (1979) supports this line of argument in his statement that one of the most difficult problems facing rehabilitation workers is their overinvolvement in the client's problems.

This explanation is further supported by the difference found between NII and MOD rehabilitation social workers. While the social workers in both these rehabilitation agencies demonstrated a similarity in the frequency dimension of the personal involvement scale, in the intensity dimension the NII social workers were not significantly different from the MOD rehabilitation social workers of the welfare agency workers.

A possible explanation for this finding is the wide variety of the clients dealt with by NII rehabilitation social workers. This may reduce somewhat the intensity of personal involvement felt by workers who focus on different kinds of loss (Eldar, 1981). A second explanation may lie in the policy differences between the two institutions: NII policy is to limit the availability of vocational rehabilitation services while in the MOD, the availability of the services is unlimited and indefinite throughout the life of the client. The results indeed suggest that worker burnout is influenced by a variety of factors acting simultaneously (e.g., the type of target population, job setting characteristics and auxiliary help available to the worker in coping with job pressures).

Further analysis showed that the five factors related to job setting differentiated significantly between the research groups (see Table 2). These findings correspond with other studies which emphasized that organizational variables influence burnout no less than psychological variables (Cherniss, 1980a, 1980b; Edelwich, 1980; Pines, Aronson & Kafry, 1981).

In evaluating job setting variables, several differences between the research groups were found. NII workers also devoted the least amount of time to supervision and were the least satisfied with it. The social welfare agency workers indicated their dissatisfaction with supervision, yet it is possible that they were compensated in the high percentage of time devoted to staff consultation relative to the NII social workers. The MOD rehabilitation social workers in contrast, reported a high percentage of time devoted to supervision and that they were relatively satisfied with it. This might be a possible element in the low burnout level expressed in the intensity dimension of the personal accomplishment scale.

It is interesting to note that the MOD rehabilitation social workers, dealing with disabled veterans, reported the heaviest caseload and the greatest feeling of bureaucratic intervention. This might be expected to increase the burnout level in the personal involvement factor, yet the results show the opposite. The explanation for this finding may lie in the mutual simultaneous influence of several variables: the high percentage of time devoted to supervision and the high level of satisfaction with it, apparently moderate the influence of the caseload burden and the feeling of bureaucratic intervention. Another possible complementary explanation may lie in the "Halo Effect" prevalent in Israeli society that disabled veterans are "heroes to be admired" (Florian, 1978; Shurka & Katz, 1976). This could be an important element which might influence workers' feelings when dealing with these veterans.

In summary, it is apparent that the sources of burnout cannot be evaluated on a one-dimensional study of a particular variable such as the type of client population but rather require systematic investigations of a variety of variables and factors that contribute to the phenomenon of professional burnout. From the above it may be concluded that burnout is a factor in most rehabilitation settings and that it must be further studied in order to discover ways of mitigating the negative effects of this phenomenon. Any attempt at combatting burnout must take into account job setting variables such as the type of clients dealt with, the caseload, frequency of supervision, satisfaction with supervision, and feeling of bureaucratic intervention.

REFERENCES

Alexy, W. (1980). Coping with loss: The principal theme postulate. *Rehabilitation Literature, 41*(3-4), 66-71.
Cherniss, C. (1980a). *Professional burnout in human service organizations*. New York: Prager Publishers.
Cherniss, C. (1980b). *Staff burnout: Job stress and the human services*. CA: Sage Publishing Inc.
Cherniss, C. & Egnatios, E. (1978). Clinical supervision in community mental health. *Social Work, 23*, 219-223.
Daley, M. R. (1979). Burnout: Smoldering problem in protective services. *Social Work, 24*(5), 375-379.
Edelwich, J. & Brodsky, A. (1980). *Burnout: Stages of disillusionment in the helping professions*. New York: Human Sciences Press.
Eldar, E. (1981). Burnout among nurses in general hospital. Tel Aviv University, MA thesis.
Emener, W. G. (1979). Professional burnout: Rehabilitation's hidden handicap. *Journal of Rehabilitation*, 53-58.
Emener, W. G. & Luck, R. S.(1980). *Emener Luck Burnout Scale* (E.L.B.O.S.).
Emener, W. G., Luck, R. S. & Gohs, F. X. (1982). A theoretical investigation of the construct burnout. *Rehabilitation Administration, 6*(4), 188-196.
Etzion, D., Kafry, D. & Pines, A. (1982). Tedium among managers: A cross-cultural American-Israeli comparison. *Journal of Psychology and Judaism, 7*(1).
Faffer, J. I. (1981). Casework with the chronically ill: A population that does not "Get Better." *Social Casework, 62*(6), 372-376.
Falek, A. & Britton, S. (1974). Phases in coping: The hypothesis and its implications. *Social Biology, 21*(1), 1-7.
Florian, V. & Shurka, E. (1986). Burnout phenomena experienced by work instructors in sheltered and rehabilitation workshops. *Journal of Applied Rehabilitation Counseling*, in press.
Florian, V. (1978). Employers' opinion of the disabled person as worker. *Rehabilitation Counseling Bulletin, 22*, 38-43.

Freudenberger, H. J. (1980). *Burnout: The high cost of high achievement.* Garden City, NY: Doubleday.

Hughes, F. (1980). Reaction to loss: Coping with disability and death. *Rehabilitation Counseling Bulletin, 24*(3).

Kafry, D. & Pines, A. (1980). The experience of tedium in life and work. *Human Relations, 33*(7), 477-503.

Kahn, R. L. (1973). Conflict, ambiguity and overload: Three elements in job stress. *Occupational Mental Health, 3*, 2-9.

Katz, S., Shurka, E. & Florian, V. (1978). The relationship between physical disability, social perception and psychological stress. *The Scandinavian Journal of Rehabilitation Medicine, 10*, 109-113.

Lattansi, M. E. (1981). Coping with work-related issues. *Personnel and Guidance Journal, 59*, 350-351.

Lewiston, N. J., Conley, J. & Blessing-Moore, J. (1981). Measurement of hypothetical burnout in cystic fibrosis caregivers. *Acta Paediatrica Scandinavica, 70*, 935-939.

Maslach, C. (1978). The client role in staff burnout. *Journal of Social Issues, 34*(4), 112-124.

Maslach, C. (1979). The burnout syndrome and patient care. In G. A. Garfield (ed.), *Stress and survival: The emotional realities of life threatening illness.* St. Louis: C.V. Mosby.

Maslach, C. (1982). *Burnout—The cost of caring.* NJ: Prentice-Hall Inc.

Maslach, C. & Jackson, S. E. (1981). The measurement of experienced burnout. *Journal of Occupational Behavior, 2*(2), 99-113.

Maslach, C. & Jackson, S. E. (1982). Burnout in health professions: A social-psychological analysis. In: G. Sanders & J. Suls (eds.), *Social psychology of health and illness.* Hillsdale, NJ: Lawrence Erlbaum.

Meadow, K. P. (1981). Burnout in professionals working with deaf children. *American Annals of the Deaf, 126*(1), 13-22.

Orfirer, A. P. (1970). Loss and sexual function in the male. In B. Shoenberg (ed.), *Loss and grief: Psychological management in medical practice.* New York: Columbia University Press.

Parkes, C. M. (1975). Psycho-Social transitions: Comparison between the reaction to loss of a limb and loss of a spouse. *British Journal of Psychiatry, 127*, 204-210.

Pines, A., Aronson, E., with Kafry, D. (1981). *Burnout: From tedium to personal growth.* New York: Macmillan Publishing, Inc.

Riggar, T. F., Harrington-Godley, S. & Hafer, M. (1984). Burnout and job satisfaction in rehabilitation administrators and divert service providers. *Rehabilitation Counseling Bulletin, 27*(3), 151-160.

Sarata, B. P. V. (1972). Job satisfaction of individual working with the mentally retarded. Ph.D. Dissertation, Yale University.

Shurka, E. & Katz, S. (1976). Evaluations of persons with a disability. The influence of disability context and personal responsibility for the disability. *Rehabilitation Psychology, 23*(3), 65-71.

Stevens, M. J. & Pfost, K. S. (1983). A problem-solving approach to staff burnout in rehabilitation settings. *Rehabilitation Counseling Bulletin, 27*(2).

Valle, S. K. (1979). Burnout: Occupational hazard for counselors. *Alcohol Health and Research World, 3*, 10-14.

Wright, B. A. (1983). *Physical disability: A psychosocial approach.* 2nd ed. New York: Harper & Row Publishers.

Burnout Research in the Social Services: A Critique

Christina Maslach

SUMMARY. The six articles in this special issue on burnout are critically reviewed. The shortcomings of these articles, both conceptual and empirical, limit the contributions that this special issue can make to our understanding of burnout.

The phenomenon of burnout first became the subject of public attention in the mid-1970s (Freudenberger, 1974, 1975; Maslach, 1976). Since that time, there has been a wealth of writing on this topic, including numerous books, pamphlets, and articles in both scholarly journals and popular magazines. Some of this writing has focused on burnout within a particular profession (such as teaching, nursing, social work), while some of it has considered burnout as it occurs across a wide range of human service, caregiving occupations. Some authors have tried to grapple with the issue of what causes burnout to occur, while others have proposed various ways of dealing with it. Many interesting ideas and issues have been raised, as well as suggested solutions for the problems posed by burnout. What characterizes much of the burnout literature, particularly in its early years, is that most of it was not based on any empirical research. For example, a review of most of the existing literature through 1981 found that only about 15% of the publications involved systematic data collection (Maslach, 1982a). Thus, while there was

Dr. Maslach is Associate Professor of Psychology, Department of Psychology, University of California, Berkeley, CA 94720.

much speculation (and even dogmatic statements) about what burnout is and what should be done about it, there was very little hard evidence to test the truth of these assertions.

Happily, the trend in recent years has been one of increased research activity. More and more often, published articles on burnout present a systematic study of hypotheses, using well-developed measures and sophisticated data analyses. As later studies replicate, extend, and build upon the findings of the earlier ones, we will gain a greater understanding of burnout and be able to develop more comprehensive models of the burnout phenomenon. Moreover, we will acquire a more solid knowledge base for recommendations concerning intervention and change.

The work on burnout in the social services mirrors the trends in the burnout field as a whole. Clearly, burnout has been an important issue in social services, judging from the number of workshops and professional meetings organized around this topic. However, systematic research on burnout has gotten underway only recently. Thus, it is a landmark event to have an entire issue of the *Journal of Social Service Research* devoted to theoretical and empirical work on burnout. Because of this, the articles in this issue take on a special status. Not only do they represent the "state of the art" in social service research on burnout, but they may serve as a model for future studies. The potential impact of their prominent position makes it imperative that they be scrutinized carefully and evaluated critically. This has been my task as the discussant for this issue.

CONTRIBUTIONS OF THE SPECIAL ISSUE

The six articles in this issue consist of five research studies and one literature review. The review paper (Courage & Williams) provides a useful listing of many possible factors in the burnout syndrome, and categorizes them in terms of three dimensions: provider, recipient, and organization. In a sense, these are the "pieces" in the burnout puzzle—or at least the pieces that have been identified so far. What the missing pieces are, and more importantly, how the pieces are put together to provide a complete picture of burnout, are important challenges for future theory and research.

The five studies differ somewhat in the variables they assess, but they share several characteristics. Most of the studies are correlational in design, with the exception of the study comparing specific groups of social workers (Stav, Florian & Shurka). They all involve questionnaire surveys, three of which were conducted by mail, and thus they rely exclusively on self-report data. In all cases, burnout was assessed by the same research measure, the Maslach Burnout Inventory (MBI), thus providing some comparability between the studies. All of the respondents were social workers, albeit with varying specializations and job responsibilities. Most of these workers were female; two of the samples were exclusively female. Of the four American samples, three were from the middle regions of the country. The one national American sample (Himle, Jayaratne & Chess) represents a rarity in the burnout literature, in which local samples are the norm. Also exceptional in this regard is the Israeli sample (Stav, Florian & Shurka), given that the majority of burnout studies have been conducted with American subjects.

Each of these five studies takes a different approach to the investigation of burnout. The work by LeCroy and Rank is the most broad in scope, focusing on both personal and job-related variables, as well as on coping mechanisms. Attention to both personal and job factors also characterizes two other studies, although the researchers differ most noticeably in the personal variables they chose to assess. In one case, the focus was on the personal outcome variable of psychological strain (Himle, Jayaratne & Chess), while in the other, the focus was on a presumably causal personality variable (Johnson & Stone). A narrower focus on just job setting factors was taken by Stav, Florian and Shurka, while the study by Corcoran dealt with only one job-related variable – the worker's perceptions of clients.

Overall, the pattern of reported results is consistent with those presented in other published studies. Higher levels of experienced burnout were associated with more negative ratings of certain aspects of the work environment: autonomy, comfort, challenge, client contact, and coworker support. Burnout was also associated with lower job satisfaction and greater intention to quit the job. At the personal level, burnout was related to lower levels of self-esteem, lower use of coping mechanisms, more hassles in one's daily life, and lower scores on Type A personality style. In general, both negative environment and negative personal factors are linked to burnout—although the causal nature of these linkages is not at all clear. Moreover, it is not clear whether these particular environmental and personal variables are indeed the most important and relevant ones with respect to burnout.

Although this general summary, and the conclusions of the authors, often refer to burnout as a unitary phenomenon, it is important to note that it is actually a multidimensional construct. Burnout is defined as a syndrome of emotional exhaustion, depersonalization, and reduced personal accomplishment that can occur among individuals who do "people-work" of some kind, and the MBI (which was utilized in all of the studies in this issue) was specifically designed to assess these three components of burnout (Maslach & Jackson, 1981, 1986). What has been emerging in current research (and is borne out by the studies in this issue) is that these three components of burnout are differentially related to other variables (Maslach & Jackson, 1984). Certain job factors may be predictive of emotional exhaustion, but not of the other aspects of burnout, while other factors are predictive of reduced personal accomplishment, or depersonalization. Similarly, these three components of burnout are differentially related to various outcomes. Given the accumulating evidence for the multidimensional nature of burnout, it is important that researchers take this into account in their theorizing about the burnout syndrome. The variables to be chosen for study should be conceptualized in terms of their hypothesized relationship with one or more of the burnout components, and these hypotheses should then be tested directly.

SHORTCOMINGS OF THE SPECIAL ISSUE

While there are potential gains from all six of these articles, there are also problems, both conceptual and empirical, with the set of articles in this issue. The problems limit the conclusions we can draw, and the understanding we can achieve, about the phenomenon of burnout.

Conceptual Problems

What is striking about the entire issue is the conceptual weakness that occurs throughout. There are not clearly articulated views about what burnout is, what might be its causes and outcomes, or how to go about investigating it. This is not to say that all researchers should agree on a particular theoretical approach—at this early stage in burnout research, a diversity of competing viewpoints is to be expected, and even welcomed. However, it should be the case that there is conceptual clarity within each research study—clarity as to definition, research rationale, and interpretation of findings.

Definitional issues. Definitions of burnout are many and varied, a state of affairs that has important implications for the progress of burnout research (Maslach, 1982b). However, in terms of any one study, the task for the researcher is to choose a particular definition, develop a set of relevant working hypotheses, and use measures that are consistent with that definition. This definitional task is not handled well by the researchers represented in the special issue. None of the authors provide a precise statement of how they are conceptualizing burnout. Sometimes there is no definition at all (LeCroy & Rank, Corcoran). Sometimes brief references are made to various definitions, but without choosing one to utilize in the study (Himle et al., Stav et al.). Sometimes a general definition is given, but without acknowledging the source of that definition or (if the definition is original to the authors) indicating the theoretical rationale underlying it (Courage & Rank, Johnson & Stone). The Johnson & Stone article is particularly murky with respect to definition, because the authors first state that Freudenberger and Maslach "coined" the term of burnout, then give a definition that is not that of either Freudenberger or Maslach (and which is unattributed to anyone else), and then equate burnout with the more general construct of "job stress" (an equation that is highly questionable, conceptually). It should be noted that burnout is not the only construct that is poorly defined in these studies—many of the other variables are not well conceptualized (beyond the operational definition of the measure used to assess them).

Theoretical issues. Related to the general lack of definition is a lack of theoretical frameworks for the studies. No conceptual models of burnout are presented, from which a set of hypotheses can be derived and then tested. There are no clearly stated guiding ideas or underlying rationales for the design and method of the research. In many cases, the authors select certain variables to study but without explaining why they should be important or how they should be related to burnout. For example, the conceptual rationale for studying gender and burnout is never made clear, beyond referring to weak and inconsistent findings in past research (Corcoran, Himle et al.). Different groups of Israeli social workers are hypothesized to differ in burnout, but no reasons are given for this prediction or for the possible role of "job setting" factors (Stav et al.). Likewise, no theoretical rationale is presented for the decision to assess personal hassles and Type A personality (Johnson & Stone). This is not to say that all of these variables are unworthy of study— to the contrary, they may indeed be very important factors in the burnout phenomenon. However, there should be some persuasive reasons underlying the choice of these variables, and these reasons should be clearly articulated by the authors.

The atheoretical tone of the studies makes them appear to be "fishing expeditions," in which the researcher simply throws out a questionnaire net and sees what results turn up in it. Such an unguided search makes interpretation of the findings (or the lack of them) a difficult task. Are the results supportive of any of the authors' ideas about burnout, or not? To what extent are the results due purely to chance (a likely explanation when many variables are assessed and only a few significant results emerge)? Are there important inconsistencies or contradictions with other work in the field? What is the meaning of a lack of significant findings—incorrect hypothesis? methodological problem? chance? Questions such as these are not always easy to answer, but they are especially problematic for studies that are not grounded in a theoretical framework. If we cannot arrive at any clear understanding of the data, then the studies cannot make much of a contribution to the field.

Theoretical issues are also a problem for the review article (Courage & Rank), particularly because the authors claim to be presenting a new approach to studying burnout. While they do propose three dimensions and then specify a number of variables on each of these dimensions, they say nothing clear about how all of this is related to burnout (other than some vague references to "balance" and "optimal" relationships). There is no theoretical rationale for putting these dimensions together into a cube, nor a persuasive argument as to the merits of doing so. For example, how does an understanding of the burnout process arise from this structural approach? How can new hypotheses and predicted relationships actually be generated from this cube? What is the advantage of looking at individual "cells" (which contain only one variable from each dimension) when most situations would actually be characterized by all variables? What are the proposed relationships between variables within one dimension? What is the theoretical purpose of studies which vary each of the variables on one dimension with each of the variables on the second dimension while holding the third dimension constant? How could such studies even be done? Contrary to the authors' assertions, these and many other questions are not answered in their article. While they have generated a list of variables that are potentially relevant to burnout, they have not developed a theoretical framework for understanding this phenomenon.

A problem that may be related, at least in part, to these issues of conceptual fuzziness is the apparent failure to do thorough reviews of the literature. Some of the authors do not seem to be familiar with much of the published work that is relevant to their study, particularly work outside the field of social services. While it is true that the burnout literature is not neatly centralized within a few journals, but is scattered across a wide variety of them, it is also the case that there are many resources to aid the researcher in surveying the field, including computerized library searches and books with extensive reference lists. Research can be improved via knowledge of other studies that have addressed similar or related questions, and via critical analysis of both their flaws and virtues.

Empirical Problems

Aside from the conceptual problems in this special issue, the research studies suffer from a number of empirical difficulties that limit the significance of their contribution. These include problems with subject samples, measurement, and analysis of the results.

Subject samples. The social worker samples reported in these studies vary considerably in size and selection procedure. Problems of self-selection and of insufficient sample size for the number of variables studied occur in varying degrees (but are most acute for the Johnson & Stone study). It is not always clear how representative these samples are of the larger population of social workers, although the most representative seem to be the national American sample (Himle et al.) and the national Israeli sample (Stav et al.). None of the studies provides a sufficient description about the initial information subjects were given about the research (e.g., what did they think the study was about? and was burnout mentioned specifically?). The subjects' expectations or "mind-set" could have influenced the way they responded to questions.

Measurement. There are many issues to be raised with the measurement procedures used in these studies. First, too little is usually said about the measures used. There need to be a clearer statement about the conceptual variable that is being assessed, the number and type of items (providing a sample item is often helpful), and the method of scoring items and computing total scores. Psychometric analyses that have been published elsewhere can be referenced, and need not be repeated in the text. However, any measures that lack such prior psychometric work need to be evaluated for reliability and validity by the authors, and the results of these analyses should appear in the article. For example, more psychometric analyses should have been done for the Jourard Impression Scale, especially because it was the major dependent measure in the study (Corcoran).

Second, as a co-author of the MBI, I was particularly distressed by the ways in which it was misused by the issue authors. It was not always properly referenced (Maslach & Jackson, 1981), nor was it always described accurately. It has 22 items, which are divided into three subscales: Emotional Exhaustion, Depersonalization, and Personal Accomplishment (reverse scoring). The three items to which they were referring were in the original factor analyses for the MBI, but these items did not load on any subscale and their relation to the three components of burnout was unclear. Thus, these items were deleted from the MBI, although with the recommendation that further developmental work might be pursued in this area. In the study by Corcoran, only two of the subscales were used, without any rationale for the omission of the third.

Another set of problems with the MBI has to do with the item format and scoring. Each of the items is rated in terms of frequency ("never" – "every day") and intensity ("very mild" – "very strong"). (However, it should be noted that in the new edition of the MBI, the recommendation is that the frequency rating alone is sufficient for most research purposes [Maslach & Jackson, 1986]). Whether Corcoran and LeCroy and Rank actually followed these scoring procedures is not clear from their descriptions. However, Himle et al. changed the format to a single rating of "strongly agree" – "strongly disagree," and also reduced the 9-item subscale of Emotional Exhaustion to just one item. Johnson and Stone combined the frequency and intensity ratings (despite the specific statement by Maslach & Jackson, 1981, that this should not be done), and also combined the Emotional Exhaustion and Depersonalization subscales into a single measure. If any modifications are going to be made in an established measure, then it is incumbent upon the authors to provide sufficient psychometric data to establish that such modifications do not change the measure in any substantive way. Changing the psychometric rules is not justified by a desire to merely simplify research procedures or shorten a long questionnaire. Because of the changes made by these authors, we cannot be sure about what the scores actually mean, nor can we compare the data from these studies with those collected by other researchers.

Analysis of results. A striking trend in these five studies is that the findings are generally weak, sparse, and account for very little of the variance – and yet much is made of them. For example, Himle et al. find very little evidence to support their predictions of gender differences, but they go on to propose "gender-specific interventions." Stav et al. find almost no support for their predictions of burnout differences between subgroups of rehabilitation social workers, but they then discuss intervention strategies. While Corcoran's findings support the construct validity of burnout (since negative impressions of clients are part of the definition of depersonalization), he goes beyond that to make inferences about clinical practice. LeCroy & Rank draw conclusions about a "model" of burnout, even though their study was not designed to test any model. The strongly-stated conclusion of Johnson & Stone, that "there does not appear to be a substantial relationship between stress and features of the work environment or specific aspects of the individual's personality," can *not* be made on the basis of their study, in which only 46 subjects completed just one personality measure and just one perceptual measure of work environment. Given that such a conclusion flies in the face of a great deal of work on stress, the authors should gather far more substantial research evidence before making such an extreme statement.

The studies in this issue are all cross-sectional in design, and rely exclusively on self-report data. While this is typical of most current research on burnout, there are limitations. Chief among these is the reliance on correlational data analyses, even though the major issues of interest involve questions of causal relationships. Interpretation of the correlational findings is often ambiguous as to what factor is causing what outcome. For example, Himle et al. talk about "intent to quit" as a stressor that predicts burnout—yet an equally plausible interpretation is that the causal sequence is the reverse: burnout leads to the intention to quit the job. Unfortunately, the nature of the research does not allow us to evaluate which of these alternative explanations is more correct. Longitudinal studies are a very important item on the agenda for future burnout research, as is the use of objective measures other than self-report. Fortunately, the first such study has now been completed (Jackson, Schwab & Schuler, in press), and more should be forthcoming.

CONCLUDING REMARKS

It has not been easy to present a critical evaluation of the articles in this special issue on burnout. As a researcher who has worked in this field for a long time, and who has tried hard to encourage studies of this topic, I would have liked to have been completely enthusiastic about this special issue and the contributions that it made. However, it is my firm belief that the field is only going to advance if we do the best theoretical and empirical work possible — research that is well-designed and carefully controlled, and that investigates important and meaningful questions within the context of a well-articulated theoretical framework. Thus, my comments are not meant to be criticisms of the authors, but rather constructive guidelines on how the quality of the theory and research could be improved. I know of no "perfect" studies that are without flaws and limitations (and that includes my own), but that should not stop us from striving to reach the ideal. Burnout is a problem of serious importance in the social services, as well as in other people-oriented occupations — and the goal of understanding it, and eventually ameliorating it, demands our best efforts.

REFERENCES

Freudenberger, H. J. (1974). Staff burn-out. *Journal of Social Issues, 30*(1), 159-165.
Freudenberger, H. J. (1975). The staff burnout-syndrome in alternative institutions. *Psychotherapy: Theory, Research, and Practice, 12*(1), 73-82.
Jackson, S. E., Schwab, R. L. & Schuler, R. S. (in press). Understanding the burnout phenomenon. *Journal of Applied Psychology*.
Maslach, C. (1976). Burned-out. *Human Behavior, 5*(9), 16-22.
Maslach, C. (1982a). *Burnout: The cost of caring*. Englewood Cliffs, NJ: Prentice-Hall.
Maslach, C. (1982b). Understanding burnout: Definitional issues in analyzing a complex phenomenon. In W. S. Paine (ed.), *Job stress and burnout*. Beverly Hills, CA: Sage, pp. 29-40.
Maslach, C. & Jackson, S. E. (1981). *Maslach burnout inventory*. Research ed. Palo Alto, CA: Consulting Psychologists Press.
Maslach, C. & Jackson, S. E. (1984). Burnout in organizational settings. *Applied Social Psychology Annual, 5*, 133-153.
Maslach, C. & Jackson, S. E. (1986). *Maslach burnout inventory*. 2nd ed. Palo Alto, CA: Consulting Psychologists Press.